T0362500

Pediatric Dermatology
Part II

Editor

KELLY M. CORDORO

DERMATOLOGIC CLINICS

www.derm.theclinics.com

Consulting Editor
BRUCE H. THIERS

April 2022 • Volume 40 • Number 2

ELSEVIER

1600 John F. Kennedy Boulevard • Suite 1800 • Philadelphia, Pennsylvania, 19103-2899

http://www.theclinics.com

DERMATOLOGIC CLINICS Volume 40, Number 2
April 2022 ISSN 0733-8635, ISBN-13: 978-0-323-89762-4

Editor: Katerina Heidhausen
Developmental Editor: Karen Justine Solomon

© **2022 Elsevier Inc. All rights reserved.**

This periodical and the individual contributions contained in it are protected under copyright by Elsevier, and the following terms and conditions apply to their use:

Photocopying
Single photocopies of single articles may be made for personal use as allowed by national copyright laws. Permission of the Publisher and payment of a fee is required for all other photocopying, including multiple or systematic copying, copying for advertising or promotional purposes, resale, and all forms of document delivery. Special rates are available for educational institutions that wish to make photocopies for non-profit educational classroom use. For information on how to seek permission visit www.elsevier.com/permissions or call: (+44) 1865 843830 (UK)/(+1) 215 239 3804 (USA).

Derivative Works
Subscribers may reproduce tables of contents or prepare lists of articles including abstracts for internal circulation within their institutions. Permission of the Publisher is required for resale or distribution outside the institution. Permission of the Publisher is required for all other derivative works, including compilations and translations (please consult www.elsevier.com/permissions).

Electronic Storage or Usage
Permission of the Publisher is required to store or use electronically any material contained in this periodical, including any article or part of an article (please consult www.elsevier.com/permissions). Except as outlined above, no part of this publication may be reproduced, stored in a retrieval system or transmitted in any form or by any means, electronic, mechanical, photocopying, recording or otherwise, without prior written permission of the Publisher.

Notice
No responsibility is assumed by the Publisher for any injury and/or damage to persons or property as a matter of products liability, negligence or otherwise, or from any use or operation of any methods, products, instructions or ideas contained in the material herein. Because of rapid advances in the medical sciences, in particular, independent verification of diagnoses and drug dosages should be made.

Although all advertising material is expected to conform to ethical (medical) standards, inclusion in this publication does not constitute a guarantee or endorsement of the quality or value of such product or of the claims made of it by its manufacturer.

Dermatologic Clinics (ISSN 0733-8635) is published quarterly by Elsevier Inc., 360 Park Avenue South, New York, NY 10010-1710. Months of publication are January, April, July, and October. Business and editorial offices: 1600 John F. Kennedy Blvd., Suite 1800, Philadelphia, PA 19103-2899. Customer service office: 11830 Westline Drive, St. Louis, MO 63146. Periodicals postage paid at New York, NY, and additional mailing offices. Subscription prices are USD 429.00 per year for US individuals, USD 1,035.00 per year for US institutions, USD 469.00 per year for Canadian individuals, USD 1,071.00 per year for Canadian institutions, USD 525.00 per year for international individuals, USD 1,071.00 per year for international institutions, USD 100.00 per year for US students/residents, USD 100.00 per year for Canadian students/residents, and USD 240 per year for international students/residents. International air speed delivery is included in all *Clinics* subscription prices. All prices are subject to change without notice. **POSTMASTER:** Send address changes to *Dermatologic Clinics*, Elsevier Health Sciences Division, Subscription Customer Service, 3251 Riverport Lane, Maryland Heights, MO 63043. **Customer Service: 1-800-654-2452 (U.S. and Canada); 314-447-8871 (outside U.S. and Canada). Fax: 314-447-8029. E-mail: journalscustomerservice-usa@elsevier.com (for print support); journalsonlinesupport-usa@elsevier.com (for online support).**

Reprints. For copies of 100 or more, of articles in this publication, please contact the Commercial Reprints Department, Elsevier Inc., 360 Park Avenue South, New York, New York 10010-1710. Tel.: 212-633-3874; Fax: 212-633-3820; Email: reprints@elsevier.com.

The *Dermatologic Clinics* is covered in *MEDLINE/PubMed (Index Medicus), Current Contents/Clinical Medicine, Excerpta Medica, Chemical Abstracts,* and *ISI/BIOMED.*

Contributors

CONSULTING EDITOR

BRUCE H. THIERS, MD
Professor and Chairman Emeritus, Department of Dermatology and Dermatologic Surgery, Medical University of South Carolina, Charleston, South Carolina

EDITOR

KELLY M. CORDORO, MD
Professor of Dermatology and Pediatrics, Chief, Division of Pediatric Dermatology, Fellowship Director, Pediatric Dermatology, McCalmont Family Endowed Professor in Pediatric Dermatology, Department of Dermatology, University of California, San Francisco, UCSF Benioff Children's Hospital, San Francisco, San Francisco, California

AUTHORS

SARAH D. CIPRIANO, MD, MPH, MS
Department of Dermatology, University of Utah, Salt Lake City, Utah

KELLY M. CORDORO, MD
Professor of Dermatology and Pediatrics, Chief, Division of Pediatric Dermatology, Fellowship Director, Pediatric Dermatology, McCalmont Family Endowed Professor in Pediatric Dermatology, Department of Dermatology, University of California, San Francisco, UCSF Benioff Children's Hospital, San Francisco, San Francisco, California

PAIGE K. DEKKER, MD
Georgetown University School of Medicine, Washington, DC

NATALIA M. FONTECILLA, MD
Department of Dermatology, Johns Hopkins Medicine, Baltimore, Maryland

TRACY FUNK, MD
Associate Professor of Dermatology and Pediatrics, Division Head of Pediatric Dermatology, Department of Dermatology, Oregon Health & Science University, Portland, Oregon

DEEPTI GUPTA, MD
Associate Professor, Department of Pediatrics, Division of Dermatology, Seattle Children's Hospital/University of Washington School of Medicine, Seattle, Washington

JESSICA S. HABER, MD
Ronald O. Perelman Department of Dermatology, NYU Grossman School of Medicine, NYU Langone Dermatology Associates, New York, New York

JENNIFER T. HUANG, MD
Boston Children's Hospital, Dermatology Program, Harvard Medical School, Boston, Massachusetts

DANNY W. LINGGONEGORO, BS
Boston Children's Hospital, Dermatology Program, Harvard Medical School, Boston, Massachusetts

MARY KATE LOCKHART, MD
Division of Dermatology, Department of Pediatrics, Cardinal Glennon Children's Hospital, St. Louis University School of Medicine, St Louis, Missouri

SHEILAGH M. MAGUINESS, MD
Associate Professor, Division of Pediatric Dermatology, Department of Dermatology, University of Minnesota, Minneapolis, Minnesota

DANIELLE MCCLANAHAN, MD
Department of Dermatology, Oregon Health & Science University, Portland, Oregon

REESA L. MONIR, MD
Resident, Department of Dermatology, University of Florida College of Medicine, Gainesville, Florida

NANJIBA NAWAZ, BA
Medical Student, Penn State College of Medicine, Hershey, Pennsylvania

CYNTHIA L. NICHOLSON, MD
Assistant Professor, Division of Pediatric Dermatology, Department of Dermatology, University of Minnesota, Minneapolis, Minnesota

SCOTT A. NORTON, MD, MPH, MSc
Department of Dermatology, George Washington University School of Medicine and Health Sciences, Washington, DC

JENNIFER ORNELAS, MD
Department of Dermatology, University of California, San Francisco School of Medicine, San Francisco, California

VIKASH S. OZA, MD
NYU:Ronald O. Perelman Department of Dermatology, NYU Grossman School of Medicine, NYU Langone Dermatology Associates, New York, New York

JENNIFER J. SCHOCH, MD
Associate Professor, Department of Dermatology, University of Florida College of Medicine, Gainesville, Florida

GABRIELLE H. SCHWARTZMAN, BS
Department of Dermatology, George Washington University School of Medicine and Health Sciences, Washington, DC

ELAINE C. SIEGFRIED, MD
Division of Dermatology, Department of Pediatrics, Cardinal Glennon Children's Hospital, St. Louis University School of Medicine, St Louis, Missouri

ANNA S. SILVERSTEIN, MD
University of North Carolina School of Medicine, Chapel Hill, North Carolina

ALISON SMALL, MD
Assistant Professor of Dermatology and Pediatrics, Co-Director OHSU Hemangioma and Vascular Birthmarks Clinic, Assoicate Fellowship Director of Pediatric Dermatology, Department of Dermatology, Oregon Health & Science University, Portland, Oregon

HANNAH SONG, MD
Boston Children's Hospital, Dermatology Program, Harvard Medical School, Boston, Massachusetts

RYAN M. SVOBODA, MD, MS
Dermatology Resident, Penn State/ Hershey Medical Center, Department of Dermatology, Hershey, Pennsylvania

ANDREA L. ZAENGLEIN, MD
Professor of Dermatology and Pediatrics, Penn State/ Hershey Medical Center, Departments of Dermatology and Pediatrics, Hershey, Pennsylvania

Contents

Preface: From Clinic to Hospital and Gold Standard to Substandard: The Complexities of Care of Pediatric Patients ix

Kelly M. Cordoro

Clinical Relevance of the Microbiome in Pediatric Skin Disease: A Review 117

Reesa L. Monir and Jennifer J. Schoch

The human microbiome encompasses the microorganisms that live in and on the body. During the prenatal and infantile periods, foundations for the cutaneous and gut microbiomes are being established and refined concurrently with the development of immune function. Herein, we review the relevance of the microbiome to five conditions commonly encountered in pediatric dermatology: acne, alopecia areata, atopic dermatitis, psoriasis, and seborrheic dermatitis. Understanding the role microbes play in these conditions may establish the groundwork for future therapeutic interventions.

Systemic Therapy for Vascular Anomalies and the Emergence of Genotype-Guided Management 127

Cynthia L. Nicholson and Sheilagh M. Maguiness

Improved understanding of the genetic basis of vascular anomalies has uncovered a growing need for targeted medical therapies. This is especially important for lesions not amenable to surgical interventions or interventional radiologic techniques. Recent studies and case reports have documented the effective use of tailored medical therapies in several distinct types of vascular anomalies. Sirolimus, mitogen-activated protein kinase inhibitors, and phosphoinositide 3-kinase inhibitors have emerged as potential therapies. Although this remains a growing field with significant knowledge gaps, a more optimistic outlook for patients with previously devastating impact on function and quality of life seems now within reach.

Evolving Landscape of Systemic Therapy for Pediatric Atopic Dermatitis 137

Mary Kate Lockhart and Elaine C. Siegfried

Atopic dermatitis (AD) is the most common chronic inflammatory skin disease in children. Standard-of-care treatment has been topical therapy. Oral corticosteroids are also commonly used to treat intermittent flares, despite guidelines that recommend against this practice. In 2017, the first targeted biologic agent indicated for moderate-severe AD in adults received US Food and Drug Administration approval. The success of this drug, dupilumab, filled a significant unmet medical need and inspired additional interest in new drug development. This article summarizes safe and effective use of systemic therapy for moderate-severe AD in pediatric patients, highlighting dupilumab and the most promising emerging treatments.

Clinical Decisions in Pediatric Psoriasis: A Practical Approach to Systemic Therapy 145

Jennifer Ornelas and Kelly M. Cordoro

Deciding when to start and selecting a specific systemic treatment for pediatric psoriasis patients can be a complex process involving many factors. Considerations include type of psoriasis, severity, potential genetic etiologies, comorbidities, triggering events and characteristics unique to each patient. The constellation of clinical features and drug related factors may prompt selection of a specific agent. Systemic treatments may be considered on the basis of those that are "tried and true" (acitretin, methotrexate, cyclosporine, phototherapy) and "new and novel" (the biologic agents). Conventional systemic agents have decades of use to support their safety and efficacy and may be used in very flexible ways with titration of dose when maintenance is achieved or when flares occur. Targeted biologic therapies have overall reassuring safety profiles, can be very efficacious, and require little to no lab monitoring as compared to conventional systemics. However, they can be cost prohibitive and most are administered via injection. Here, we provide data and principles guiding the approach to therapy of moderate to severe psoriasis in children and use case examples to highlight several different clinical scenarios.

Hormonal Treatment of Acne and Hidradenitis Suppurativa in Adolescent Patients 167

Ryan M. Svoboda, Nanjiba Nawaz, and Andrea L. Zaenglein

Homeostasis of the cutaneous microenvironment is complex and depends on multiple intrinsic and extrinsic factors, including the influence of hormones. Hormones exert action on the hair follicle and associated sebaceous glands via both endocrine and intracrine mechanisms. The profound impact of hormonal action on follicular homeostasis can be leveraged in the treatment of disorders, such as acne and hidradenitis suppurativa. The clinician must have an intimate knowledge of the rationale for use, mechanism of action, and possible side effects of hormonal therapy when using these agents to treat adolescents with cutaneous disease.

Sweet Syndrome in the Pediatric Population 179

Danielle McClanahan, Tracy Funk, and Alison Small

Pediatric Sweet syndrome (SS) is thought to be a hypersensitivity reaction to an underlying inflammatory or infectious state and typically is diagnosed using criteria created for adult patients. Although more studies are needed to understand the etiology and natural course of pediatric SS, guidelines for work-up and treatment have been suggested. Herein, the available literature is reviewed and guidelines summarized for the clinical evaluation and management of pediatric SS.

Morbilliform Eruptions in the Hospitalized Child 191

Jessica S. Haber, Sarah D. Cipriano, and Vikash S. Oza

Morbilliform eruptions inspire a broad and varied differential spanning across inflammatory and infectious categories. The goal of this article is to help the clinician develop an approach toward the pediatric patient with a morbilliform eruption in the emergency room or hospital setting. The authors review several high-yield clinical scenarios with a focus on recently emerging and reemerging childhood diagnoses.

Supportive Oncodermatology in Pediatric Patients 203

Danny W. Linggonegoro, Hannah Song, and Jennifer T. Huang

Cutaneous reactions to targeted therapies are varied and common. Pediatric dermatology literature is emerging on the specific types and prevalence of cutaneous reactions to targeted therapies that hone in on membrane-bound receptors, intracellular signaling targets, and antiangiogenesis agents, as well as targeted immunotherapies. Data regarding the timing, severity, and treatment algorithms are most plentiful for BRAF, MEK, and EGFR inhibitors.

Laser Surgery for Dermatologic Conditions in Pediatric Patients 215

Deepti Gupta

Laser therapy is an effective treatment that can be used in a wide range of cutaneous conditions in pediatric dermatology. It is an important tool to have in one's armamentarium. The parameters within each laser can vary greatly by the make and model of the specific laser, making it difficult to make settings generalizable. The goal of this article is to provide some general guiding principles for laser choice, theory behind laser parameter selection, and education surrounding tissue response which will guide treatment parameters.

Dermatologic Consequences of Substandard, Spurious, Falsely Labeled, Falsified, and Counterfeit Medications 227

Gabrielle H. Schwartzman, Paige K. Dekker, Anna S. Silverstein, Natalia M. Fontecilla, and Scott A. Norton

This article explores dermatologic consequences of substandard, spurious, falsely labeled, falsified, and counterfeit (SSFFC) pharmaceutical products. Many SSFFC products are neither safe nor effective, and are more likely to cause adverse events than proper preparations. The products often fail to treat disease and alleviate suffering. They also affect the health of populations by generating drug-resistant pathogens. This article reviews classification systems for SSFFC medications, provides a general overview of medical and public health problems associated with substandard medications, gives examples of dermatologic consequences of each category, and recommends steps for clinicians to take upon encountering suspected SSFFC products.

DERMATOLOGIC CLINICS

FORTHCOMING ISSUES

July 2022
Food and Drug Administration's Role in Dermatology
Markham C. Luke, *Editor*

October 2022
Vascular and Lymphatic Malformations
Lara Wine Lee and Marcelo Hochman, *Editors*

January 2023
Cutaneous Oncology Update
Stan N. Tolkachjov, *Editor*

RECENT ISSUES

January 2022
Pediatric Dermatology Part I
Kelly M. Cordoro, *Editor*

October 2021
COVID-19 and the Dermatologist
Esther E. Freeman and Devon E. McMahon, *Editors*

July 2021
Hair
Neil S. Sadick, *Editor*

SERIES OF RELATED INTEREST

Medical Clinics
https://www.medical.theclinics.com/
Pediatric Clinics
https://www.pediatric.theclinics.com/
Clinics in Plastic Surgery
https://www.plasticsurgery.theclinics.com/

THE CLINICS ARE AVAILABLE ONLINE!
Access your subscription at:
www.theclinics.com

Preface

From Clinic to Hospital and Gold Standard to Substandard: The Complexities of Care of Pediatric Patients

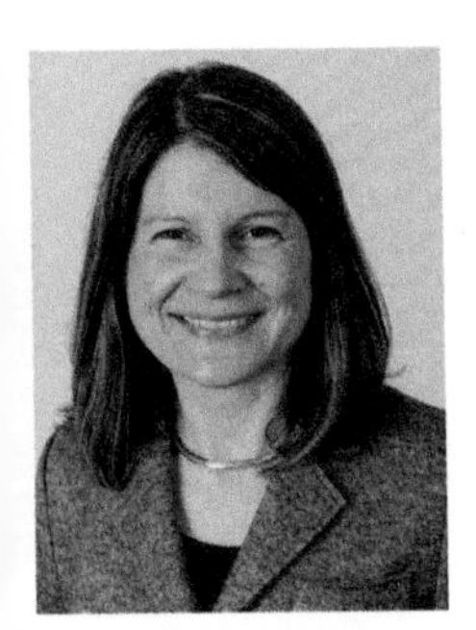

Kelly M. Cordoro, MD
Editor

Part II of *Dermatologic Clinics*: Pediatric Dermatology features a range of articles highlighting the complexities of pediatric dermatology from diagnosis to management. First, the talented lineup of experts provides a review of the microbiome in pediatric skin disease and systemic management of inflammatory skin diseases, including atopic dermatitis, psoriasis, Sweet syndrome, and acne. Then, the authors focus on the rapidly evolving state-of-the-art management of vascular malformations using genotype-guided therapies. Inpatient consultative dermatology and supportive oncodermatology in pediatric patients are two subspecialty areas that are critical to comprehensive care of hospitalized and critically ill children. These authors offer important perspectives and pearls on diagnosis and treatment of conditions observed commonly in inpatient and oncology settings, especially in the era of COVID-19 and cancer immunotherapy, respectively. Readers are then treated to an expert overview of laser surgery for dermatologic conditions in children, and the issue closes with a fascinating, deep dive into the world of counterfeit medications. These articles reflect the breadth and depth of our specialty and the multiple considerations that come to bear in medical and surgical diagnostic and therapeutic decision making for children with both complex and common skin diseases. Thank you to each of the authors for their contributions, which will elevate the care of our most vulnerable pediatric patients.

Kelly M. Cordoro, MD
UCSF Dermatology
1701 Divisadero Street
San Francisco, CA 94115, USA

E-mail address:
kelly.cordoro@ucsf.edu

Dermatol Clin 40 (2022) ix
https://doi.org/10.1016/j.det.2022.01.001
0733-8635/22/© 2022 Published by Elsevier Inc.

Clinical Relevance of the Microbiome in Pediatric Skin Disease: A Review

Reesa L. Monir, MD, Jennifer J. Schoch, MD*

KEYWORDS

• Microbiome • Pediatric • Acne • Alopecia areata • Atopic dermatitis • Eczema • Psoriasis
• Seborrheic dermatitis

KEY POINTS

- The human microbiome encompasses the microorganisms that live in and on the body, including bacteria, viruses, fungi, archaea, and mites.
- During the prenatal and infantile periods, foundations for the cutaneous and gut microbiomes are being established and refined concurrently with the development of immune function.
- Microbes and the immune system play critical roles in the pathogenesis of commonly encountered disorders in pediatric dermatology, including acne, alopecia areata, atopic dermatitis, psoriasis, and seborrheic dermatitis.
- Alterations in the microbiome are also noted during the treatment of the aforementioned disorders, suggesting a possible target for future therapeutic interventions.

INTRODUCTION

The human microbiome encompasses the microorganisms that live in and on the body. While much research focuses on bacteria, also included in this domain are viruses, fungi, archaea, and mites.[1] The microbiome is pertinent to diverse aspects of human health, from psoriasis to neonatal sepsis to cystic fibrosis.[2–4]

During the prenatal and infantile periods, all aspects of physiology are adapting and maturing in response to innate genetic predispositions and the external environment. Foundations for the cutaneous and gut microbiomes are likely established prenatally,[5] with further refinement occurring during and after birth. External factors, such as mode of delivery and method of feeding, transiently or longitudinally impact the trajectory of the microbiome.[6,7] This impressionable phase is transient, and a more stable, adult-like microbiome develops with time. The cutaneous microbiome of infants, for example, has different dominant bacteria and limited diversity that then increases and matures with time.[8] Concurrently, immune function is emerging. Microbes are crucial to the development of the immune system during the neonatal period, "teaching" it to tolerate normal flora and preventing future maladaptive inflammatory responses.[9] Both immune function and cutaneous microbes are closely involved in the development of dermatologic conditions.

Herein, we review the relevance of the microbiome to five commonly encountered pediatric skin conditions: acne, alopecia areata (AA), atopic dermatitis (AD), psoriasis, and seborrheic dermatitis. Understanding the role microbes play in these conditions will allow innovation in future therapeutic interventions.

DISCUSSION

Overview of the Microbiome

The composition of the cutaneous microbiome is determined by a number of variables, including

Department of Dermatology, University of Florida College of Medicine, 4037 NW 86th Terrace, Gainesville, FL 32606, USA
* Corresponding author.
E-mail address: jschoch@dermatology.med.ufl.edu

Dermatol Clin 40 (2022) 117–126
https://doi.org/10.1016/j.det.2021.12.001
0733-8635/22/© 2021 Elsevier Inc. All rights reserved.

anatomic location, genetics, and environmental factors.[10] A sebaceous site such as the forehead, for example, creates an environment that is hospitable to different organisms than is the dry environment of the forearm. A recent review highlighted Actinobacteria, Firmicutes, Proteobacteria, and Bacteroidetes as the dominant phyla overall in both adults and children.[11] In the gut, Firmicutes and Bacteroidetes dominate.[12] The presence of diverse microbial species is generally considered to be favorable.

Acne

Acne vulgaris is common in adults and children, and less common in infants. Clinical presentation consists of comedones, papules, pustules, and/or cysts mainly on the face, upper chest, and upper back. The condition is associated with significant morbidity, including depression, anxiety, and the potential for permanent scarring.[13] Follicular hyperkeratosis, androgenic stimulation of sebum production, inflammation, and proliferation of *Propionibacterium acnes* (now *Cutibacterium acnes*) contribute to the condition.[14]

The microbiome is central both to the pathogenesis of acne and to its treatment. *C. acnes* is the major bacterial species present in the pilosebaceous unit, accounting for nearly 90% of the bacteria in the pilosebaceous units of the nose in one study.[15] Relative abundance is similar between those with and without acne, but the presence of specific strains differs.[15] *C acnes* plays several roles in the development of acne, including increasing sebum production,[16] stimulating comedone formation,[17] and promoting inflammation.[18,19] *Malassezia* may also contribute to the disease. In a study[20] of skin surface swabs and follicular contents from inflammatory acne lesions, *Propionibacterium*, *Staphylococcus*, and *Malassezia* were noted. The amount of *Malassezia*, but not *Propionibacterium* or *Staphylococcus*, was correlated with the number of inflammatory acne lesions. In a study of preadolescent acne,[21] increasing age and increasing number of acne lesions were associated with increased *C acnes* and decreased *Streptococcus mitis*. In another smaller study of preadolescent acne,[22] all preadolescents had a predominance of *Streptococcus*, but those with acne had more *Staphylococcus* and *Propionibacterium* at all examined sites. Compared with controls, patients with acne had greater cutaneous bacterial diversity at all examined sites aside from the postauricular region. In another study, however, general loss of bacterial diversity was noted in patients with acne and correlated with disease severity.[23]

Gut dysbiosis is also seen in those with acne. In a study[24] of fecal samples, the phylum Actinobacteria was decreased in patients compared with controls, while Proteobacteria was increased. The genera *Bifidobacterium*, *Butyricicoccus*, *Coprobacillus*, *Lactobacillus*, and *Allobaculum* were decreased in those with acne relative to controls. These microbial alterations may alter the intestinal epithelial barrier and promote inflammation. The "gut–brain–skin axis" theory proposes that emotions like worry or depression alter gastrointestinal function. This, in turn, may lead to microbial dysbiosis that then contributes to inflammation locally and systemically.[25]

Microbiome alterations are also central to the treatment of acne. Treatment with isotretinoin modulates TLR2 expression to decrease the inflammatory response to *C. acnes*.[26] The effect of benzoyl peroxide, an antiinflammatory, bactericidal, and comedolytic agent, on microbial diversity is unclear. In a study of preadolescent acne,[21] treatment with benzoyl peroxide did not alter microbial diversity. In another study of preadolescent acne,[22] a decrease in microbial diversity was seen in patients with acne after treatment with both benzoyl peroxide and topical 0.025% tretinoin cream, resulting in diversity similar to what was seen in control patients. A nonsignificant decrease in the relative abundance of both *Propionibacterium* (at all examined facial sites) and *Staphylococcus* (at all sites except for the nose) was noted in preadolescents treated with benzoyl peroxide. Treatment with doxycycline was associated with an overall increase in bacterial diversity, a decrease in the relative abundance of *C. acnes,* and an increase in *Propionibacterium granulosum*.[27] The impact of doxycycline on the gut microbiome depends on the dose and duration of therapy.[28] Low doses seem to have little effect on the composition of the microbiome. Changes noted at higher doses seem to normalize after the cessation of treatment, though follow-up periods are limited. Probiotics have also shown promise in the treatment of acne.[29,30] Further studies are needed for a more complete understanding of the role the microbiome plays in acne.

Alopecia Areata

AA is a nonscarring form of hair loss most commonly involving the scalp, though potentially affecting any hair-bearing body site. Patients present with the rapid onset of single or multiple well-demarcated patches of alopecia. Disease course can be unpredictable: resolving in some, following a relapsing and remitting course in others, and becoming progressive in a small subset of patients. The most severe end of the disease spectrum includes alopecia totalis (loss of all scalp hair) and alopecia universalis (loss of all body hair).[31] Consistently effective treatments are lacking, and morbidity in pediatric patients is considerable. Children experience bullying, embarrassment, school absences, and psychiatric comorbidities, including both anxiety and depression.[32,33] The etiology of this condition is not fully understood but is thought to involve both genetic and environmental factors, including T-cell-mediated autoimmunity and loss of immune privilege in hair follicles.[34,35] Recently, the skin and gut microbiomes have been implicated in its pathogenesis.

Aberrations in the cutaneous microbiome are noted in AA. In a study[36] of the scalp microbiome, those with AA had an increased incidence of *C acnes* and a decrease in *Staphylococcus*, particularly *Staphylococcus epidermidis*, compared with the scalps of controls. Additionally, those with AA had a predominance of *Staphylococcus aureus* relative to *S. epidermidis* compared with the opposite seen in controls.

Changes in the gut microbiome are also noted in those with AA. In a study[37] of the gut microbiome in 15 patients with and 15 without alopecia universalis, bacterial species richness (known as alpha diversity) was similar between cases and controls, though the specific microbial taxa making up the microbiome differed. Those with AA had more *Parabacteroides distasonis* and *Bacteroides eggerthii*, among others. Some of the bacterial species with increased prevalence in AA have been similarly noted in gut microbiome studies of other inflammatory diseases, such as ankylosing spondylitis.[38] These bacterial shifts potentially contribute to the inflammatory environment, resulting in AA. Another possible explanation is the role of bacterial metabolic products, which can influence the development of inflammatory cells. For example, short-chain fatty acids induce the development of immune-suppressing regulatory T cells.[39] A recent review[40] on the role of micronutrients in AA noted that serum folate, vitamin D, and zinc levels tended to be lower in those with AA compared with those without AA. However, the clinical significance of these findings, including if they develop before or after the onset of alopecia, merits further research.

Striking clinical examples of the gut–skin connection in AA have been reported. In a case report of two patients with AA receiving fecal microbiota transplants for recurrent *Clostridium difficile* infections, both experienced hair regrowth following transplant.[41] One patient, after having alopecia universalis for 10 years, experienced patchy hair growth on the head and arms eight weeks following the transplant. A second patient with Crohn's disease and a 2-year history of alopecia universalis refractory to several treatments experienced hair regrowth after fecal transplant. Further research is needed to better understand the role of the microbiome in AA, particularly in the pediatric population.

Atopic Dermatitis

AD is a common childhood skin condition, with 85% of patients diagnosed before the age of five years.[42] Distribution of the pruritic, pink, scaly patches, and plaques varies with age. Infants and young children classically have involvement of face, scalp, and extensor extremities, while older children and adults have more notable involvement of the flexures. Negative consequences of the condition include chronic school absenteeism,[43] behavioral challenges,[44] and sleep disturbances,[24,25,45] among others. This condition is of particular importance given its position as the first step in the "atopic march." Skin barrier defects, inflammation, and microbial alterations seen in AD may result in subsequent food allergies, asthma, and allergic rhinitis through percutaneous sensitization to allergens.[46]

The cutaneous microbiome is of paramount importance to the pathogenesis of AD. *S. aureus* is a key player in flares, but its role in disease development remains unclear. In a study by Kennedy and colleagues[47] examining the infantile skin microbiome during the first six months of life, those who developed AD by 12 months old had significantly less colonization by commensal staphylococci, lending support to the concept of early immune tolerance preventing AD. Infants with AD were not colonized with *S. aureus* and did not have cutaneous microbial dysbiosis as is seen in older children and adults with AD. In contrast, another study[48] of infants during the first two years of life found an increased prevalence of *S. aureus* at age three months in infants who went on to develop AD. This increase was noted at the time of disease development as well as during the preceding two months. Further studies are needed to discern the role the early cutaneous microbiome plays in the development of AD.

Microbial alterations are seen at baseline and during flares in those with AD, specifically an overall decrease in bacterial diversity and overabundance of *S aureus,* that affects the inflammatory response.[49–53] A recent systematic review and meta-analysis of 95 studies found that those with AD were more likely to be colonized with *S. aureus* than were controls.[54] Disease severity and prevalence of *S. aureus* colonization were positively correlated for lesional skin sites. Patients with AD colonized by *S. aureus* not only have greater disease severity but also have increased barrier dysfunction and allergen sensitization compared with those with AD lacking *S. aureus* colonization.[55] Similar findings were noted in a study specifically examining pediatric patients.[56] Those with more severe disease had increased *S. aureus* during flares compared with those with less severe disease, in whom *S. epidermidis* predominated. Fungal and viral elements of the cutaneous microbiome were similar between groups during the study period.

Shifts in the cutaneous microbiome are noted with the treatment of AD. In a study of pediatric patients,[57] treatment of AD was associated with an increase in cutaneous bacterial diversity. Increased *S. aureus* and *S. epidermidis* were noted during flares. With treatment, increased *Corynebacterium, Propionibacterium,* and *Streptococcus* were noted. In a study of pediatric patients aged three months to five years examining the effect of topical corticosteroids alone versus topical corticosteroids and bleach baths, treatment with either regimen reestablished cutaneous microbial diversity to resemble that of controls.[52] In a study of adults,[58] treatment with topical steroids and oral antihistamines eliminated *S. aureus* from lesional and nonlesional skin in 70% of patients. Possible explanations for this change include immune alterations, skin barrier repair, or less trauma from scratching. Treatment with emollients alone similarly showed the diversification of the cutaneous microbiome, with decreased *S. aureus* following treatment.[53] Probiotics may be beneficial in the treatment and prevention of AD, but studies are still limited and conflicting.[59–61] Novel therapeutic prospects may rely on manipulating microbial alterations.

Psoriasis

Psoriasis is an inflammatory skin condition characterized by the presence of well-demarcated pink plaques with a silvery scale. Disease pathogenesis involves both genetic and environmental factors that impact innate and adaptive immunity.[62] Guttate psoriasis, presenting with many small pink scaly papules, is a variant of the classic plaque-type psoriasis which is more commonly seen in kids than in adults.[63] Pediatric psoriasis, particularly childhood guttate psoriasis, can be triggered by a preceding infection, often an oropharyngeal or perianal streptococcal infection.[63–65] A possible explanation for this association is the activation of T cells by streptococcal superantigens[66] and cross-reactivity to skin components.[67] Beyond this long-known association between microbes and psoriasis, research is now identifying a link between psoriasis and both the gut and skin microbiomes.

Gut dysbiosis is noted in patients with psoriasis. In a review of eight studies evaluating the gut microbiome in psoriasis,[68] five studies found imbalances in Firmicutes and Bacteroidetes, the two most abundant phyla in the gut microbiome. In a 100-patient study by Waldman and colleagues,[69] those with psoriasis had significantly higher levels of *Candida* in both saliva and fecal samples than did controls. The increased prevalence of psoriasis seen in those with Crohn's disease as well as the association between psoriasis and periodontal disease further suggests a gut–psoriasis connection.[70,71] As hypothesized with AA, microbial alterations may lead to disease via altered metabolism and metabolic products.[68] Alternatively, gut microbiome changes may alter immune function and the inflammatory response, as shown in murine models.[72] Treatment with secukinumab is associated with significant alterations in the gut microbiome, specifically decreased Bacteroidetes and Firmicutes and increased relative abundance of Proteobacteria.[73] Interestingly, the baseline gut microbiomes differed significantly between treatment responders and nonresponders, suggesting that the gut microbiome plays a role in treatment efficacy. Treatment with ustekinumab was not associated with any significant changes in the gut microbiome.

The cutaneous microbiome in psoriasis also differs from that of controls. In a study examining skin biopsies,[74] both those with and without psoriasis had skin predominated by Firmicutes (mainly *Staphylococci* and *Streptococci*), followed by Proteobacteria and Actinobacteria. Relative to controls, patients with psoriasis had a greater abundance of Proteobacteria and a lower abundance of Actinobacteria, with increased *Streptococci* and decreased *Staphylococci*. In a study[4] evaluating the cutaneous microbiome using skin swabs, Firmicutes were the most abundant phylum in lesions of psoriasis compared with Actinobacteria for nonlesional and control skin. Lesions of psoriasis had less *Propionibacterium* relative to nonlesional skin, which had less than control skin. *Streptococcus* was increased in lesional compared with nonlesional skin. In another study using skin swabs,[75] those with psoriasis had more diverse and heterogenous skin microbiomes than did those without psoriasis. Contrary to the aforementioned study using skin biopsies,[74] relative enrichment of *Staphylococcus aureus* was noted in both lesional and nonlesional skin of those with psoriasis, while *Staphylococcus epidermidis* and *Cutibacterium acnes* were decreased in lesional compared with healthy skin. Several other studies report increased *Staphylococcus aureus* in lesional skin along with more toxigenic strains.[76,77] Detection of these toxigenic strains correlates with disease activity, similar to what is seen in AD.[78] In susceptible individuals, breakdown of immune tolerance to cutaneous microbes may lead to the development of psoriasis via the activation of the immune system.[79] Alternatively, the differences in the cutaneous microbiome between cases and controls may relate to increased antimicrobial peptides in psoriasis.

Specifically in the pediatric population, Chen and colleagues[80] examined the impact of infection and antibiotic exposure on the future development of psoriasis in 1527 patients. Skin bacterial and viral infections, as well as fungal infections during the first two years of life, were associated with psoriasis, but exposure to systemic antibiotics was not. Another study[81] had similar findings, with infections associated with pediatric psoriasis. In a murine study,[82] neonates treated with antibiotics targeting gram-negative and gram-positive bacteria showed dysbiosis in gut and skin flora as adults, and were more susceptible to experimental psoriasis. Interestingly, adult mice treated with these same antibiotics showed decreased susceptibility to experimental psoriasis. Both findings were mediated by altered immune reactivity, including T cells and inflammatory cytokines. In another study, newborn mice with skin colonized by *S. aureus* showed a strong Th17 response that was not seen in mice colonized with *S. epidermidis*.[75] Additional research is needed to better understand the role of alterations in cutaneous flora play in psoriasis.

Seborrheic Dermatitis

Seborrheic dermatitis presents with erythema and greasy white–yellow scale or crust in areas of high sebaceous gland concentration, including the face, scalp, postauricular region, and intertriginous areas. The condition is common both in infancy and from adolescence through adulthood. In infants, the condition is commonly limited to the scalp (hence the colloquial term "cradle cap")

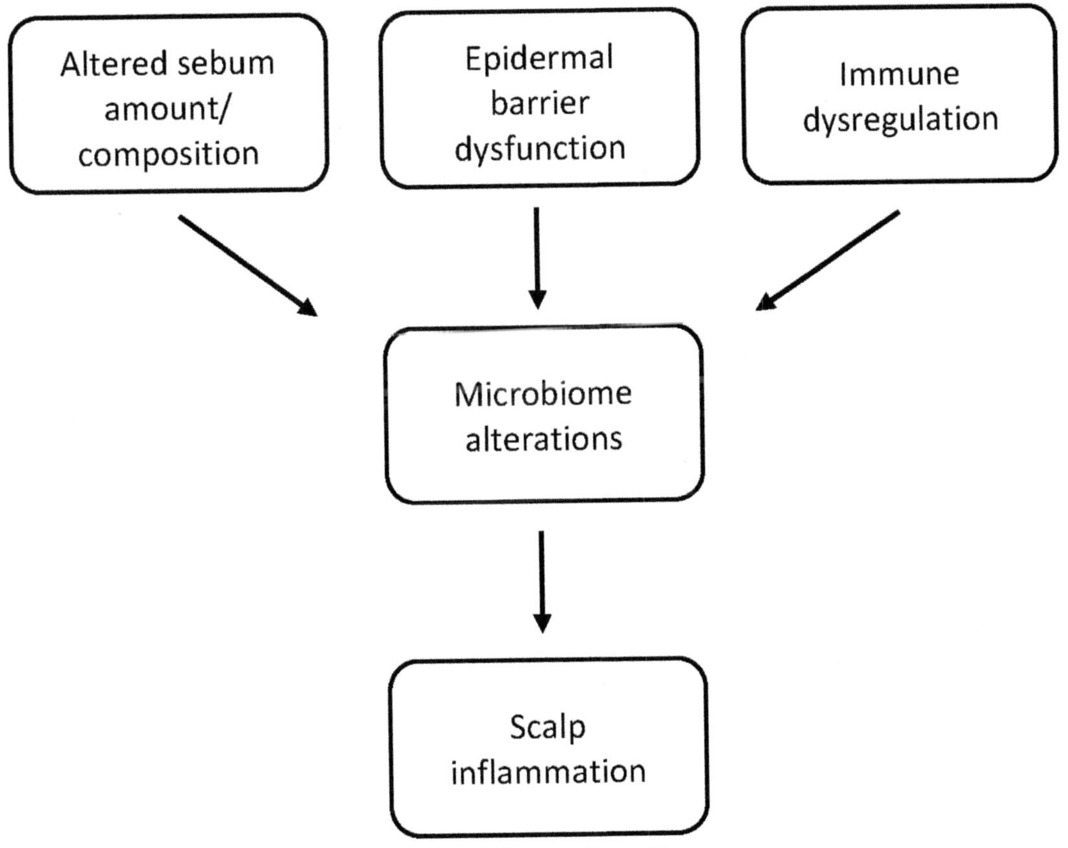

Fig. 1. Proposed model for the pathogenesis of seborrheic dermatitis.

though can be more widespread and overlap with AD.[83] Altered sebum production, host immune factors, and microbes contribute to disease development.

Bacterial and fungal dysbiosis is noted in those with seborrheic dermatitis. Studies show an increased incidence of *Malassezia* (specifically *Malassezia restricta* in some studies) and *Staphylococcal* species on the scalps of those with seborrheic dermatitis, both in adults and in infants.[84–88] Some studies also show decreased *C. acnes* in affected individuals.[85,86] The precise role these microbiome changes play, however, remains unknown. Previously, an abundance of *Malassezia* was thought to directly cause the condition because antifungals are an effective therapy, and the amount of *Malassezia* on the scalp decreases with treatment.[89–91] However, a recent review[92] of disease pathogenesis suggests that predisposing host factors, including altered sebum amount or composition, epidermal barrier dysfunction, or immune dysregulation, are the initial triggers. These alterations may then lead to microbiome changes, which in turn cause scalp inflammation and the clinical presentation of seborrheic dermatitis (**Fig. 1**). *Malassezia*, a lipophilic yeast that thrives in a sebum-rich environment, may be overrepresented in those with seborrheic dermatitis due to aberrant sebum production.[93] In infants, maternal androgens are thought to promote disease by increasing sebaceous gland activity.[94] Sebum excretion rates are highly correlated between mother and baby during the perinatal period, with rates in infants then decreasing postnatally until puberty.[95]

Notable clinical differences between pediatric patients and adults with seborrheic dermatitis suggest that etiologic differences may exist as well. In contrast to the chronic, relapsing-remitting nature of adult seborrheic dermatitis, infantile seborrheic dermatitis is usually self-limited, resolving by eight to twelve months of age in most patients.[31] Infants may also respond to more conservative treatments than are needed in adults. In addition to topical ketoconazole or topical corticosteroids, those with mild disease may respond to more frequent bathing and shampooing.[14] Future studies are required to better understand the role of the cutaneous microbiome in seborrheic dermatitis.

SUMMARY

The microbiome is pertinent to the most commonly treated pediatric dermatologic conditions, from acne to seborrheic dermatitis. Therapeutic strategies related to the microbiome are slowly being uncovered. Current research on the skin microbiome largely consists of adult subjects. Given the evolution of both the microbiome and the immune system in infants and children, this population may be a promising focus for future studies.

CLINICS CARE POINTS

- *C. acnes* contributes to the development of acne by increasing sebum production, stimulating comedone formation, and promoting inflammation, with relative abundance being similar in those with and without acne but the presence of specific strains differing.
- Gut microbiome alterations are associated with AA, which may contribute to the inflammatory environment or impact bacterial metabolic products that then influence the development of inflammatory cells.
- Flares of AD are associated with a decrease in bacterial diversity and an overabundance of *S. aureus*, but treatment restores balance to the microbiome.
- Pediatric psoriasis, particularly childhood guttate psoriasis, can be triggered by a preceding infection, possibly via immune activation and cross-reactivity to skin components.
- Altered sebum amount or composition, epidermal barrier dysfunction, or immune dysregulation are likely the initial triggers of seborrheic dermatitis which then lead to microbiome changes that cause scalp inflammation.

DISCLOSURE

The authors have no relevant conflicts of interest to disclose.

REFERENCES

1. Kong HH. Skin microbiome: genomics-based insights into the diversity and role of skin microbes. Trends Mol Med 2011;17(6):320–8. https://doi.org/10.1016/j.molmed.2011.01.013.
2. Huang YJ, LiPuma JJ. The microbiome in cystic fibrosis. Clin Chest Med 2016;37(1):59–67. https://doi.org/10.1016/j.ccm.2015.10.003.
3. Shaw AG, Sim K, Randell P, et al. Late-onset bloodstream infection and perturbed maturation of the gastrointestinal microbiota in premature infants. PLoS One 2015;10(7):e0132923. https://doi.org/10.1371/journal.pone.0132923.

4. Gao Z, hong TC, Strober BE, et al. Substantial alterations of the cutaneous bacterial biota in psoriatic lesions. PLoS One 2008;3(7):e2719. https://doi.org/10.1371/journal.pone.0002719.
5. Jiménez E, Fernández L, Marín ML, et al. Isolation of commensal bacteria from umbilical cord blood of healthy neonates born by cesarean section. Curr Microbiol 2005;51(4):270–4. https://doi.org/10.1007/s00284-005-0020-3.
6. Brink LR, Mercer KE, Piccolo BD, et al. Neonatal diet alters fecal microbiota and metabolome profiles at different ages in infants fed breast milk or formula. Am J Clin Nutr 2020;111(6):1190–202. https://doi.org/10.1093/ajcn/nqaa076.
7. Dominguez-Bello MG, Costello EK, Contreras M, et al. Delivery mode shapes the acquisition and structure of the initial microbiota across multiple body habitats in newborns. Proc Natl Acad Sci U S A 2010;107(26):11971–5. https://doi.org/10.1073/pnas.1002601107.
8. Capone KA, Dowd SE, Stamatas GN, et al. Diversity of the human skin microbiome early in life. J Invest Dermatol 2011;131(10):2026–32. https://doi.org/10.1038/jid.2011.168.
9. Scharschmidt TC. Establishing tolerance to commensal skin bacteria: timing is everything. Dermatol Clin 2017;35(1):1–9. https://doi.org/10.1016/j.det.2016.07.007.
10. Grice EA, Segre JA. The skin microbiome. Nat Rev Microbiol 2011;9(4):244–53. https://doi.org/10.1038/nrmicro2537.
11. Schoch JJ, Monir RL, Satcher KG, et al. The infantile cutaneous microbiome: a review. Pediatr Dermatol 2019;36(5):574–80. https://doi.org/10.1111/pde.13870.
12. Arumugam M, Raes J, Pelletier E, et al. Enterotypes of the human gut microbiome. Nature 2011;473(7346):174–80. https://doi.org/10.1038/nature09944.
13. Samuels DV, Rosenthal R, Lin R, et al. Acne vulgaris and risk of depression and anxiety: a meta-analytic review. J Am Acad Dermatol 2020;83(2):532–41. https://doi.org/10.1016/j.jaad.2020.02.040.
14. Bolognia JL, Schaffer JV, Cerroni L. Dermatology. 4th edition. Elsevier; 2018. Available at: https://www.us.elsevierhealth.com/dermatology-2-volume-set-9780702062759.html. March 13, 2021.
15. Fitz-Gibbon S, Tomida S, Chiu BH, et al. Propionibacterium acnes strain populations in the human skin microbiome associated with acne. J Invest Dermatol 2013;133(9):2152–60. https://doi.org/10.1038/jid.2013.21.
16. Iinuma K, Sato T, Akimoto N, et al. Involvement of propionibacterium acnes in the augmentation of lipogenesis in hamster sebaceous glands in vivo and in vitro. J Invest Dermatol 2009;129(9):2113–9. https://doi.org/10.1038/jid.2009.46.
17. Burkhart CG, Burkhart CN. Expanding the microcomedone theory and acne therapeutics: propionibacterium acnes biofilm produces biological glue that holds corneocytes together to form plug. J Am Acad Dermatol 2007;57(4):722–4. https://doi.org/10.1016/j.jaad.2007.05.013.
18. Li ZJ, Choi DK, Sohn KC, et al. Propionibacterium acnes activates the NLRP3 inflammasome in human sebocytes. J Invest Dermatol 2014;134(11):2747–56. https://doi.org/10.1038/jid.2014.221.
19. Kim J, Ochoa MT, Krutzik SR, et al. Activation of toll-like receptor 2 in acne triggers inflammatory cytokine responses. J Immunol 2002;169(3):1535–41. https://doi.org/10.4049/jimmunol.169.3.1535.
20. Akaza N, Akamatsu H, Numata S, et al. Microorganisms inhabiting follicular contents of facial acne are not only Propionibacterium but also Malassezia spp. J Dermatol 2016;43(8):906–11. https://doi.org/10.1111/1346-8138.13245.
21. Ahluwalia J, Borok J, Haddock ES, et al. The microbiome in preadolescent acne: assessment and prospective analysis of the influence of benzoyl peroxide. Pediatr Dermatol 2019;36(2):200–6. https://doi.org/10.1111/pde.13741.
22. Coughlin CC, Swink SM, Horwinski J, et al. The preadolescent acne microbiome: a prospective, randomized, pilot study investigating characterization and effects of acne therapy. Pediatr Dermatol 2017;34(6):661–4. https://doi.org/10.1111/pde.13261.
23. Dagnelie MA, Montassier E, Khammari A, et al. Inflammatory skin is associated with changes in the skin microbiota composition on the back of severe acne patients. Exp Dermatol 2019;28(8):961–7. https://doi.org/10.1111/exd.13988.
24. Yan HM, Zhao HJ, Guo DY, et al. Gut microbiota alterations in moderate to severe acne vulgaris patients. J Dermatol 2018;45(10):1166–71. https://doi.org/10.1111/1346-8138.14586.
25. Bowe WP, Logan AC. Acne vulgaris, probiotics and the gut-brain-skin axis - back to the future? Gut Pathog 2011;3(1):1. https://doi.org/10.1186/1757-4749-3-1.
26. Dispenza MC, Wolpert EB, Gilliland KL, et al. Systemic isotretinoin therapy normalizes exaggerated TLR-2-mediated innate immune responses in acne patients. J Invest Dermatol 2012;132(9):2198–205. https://doi.org/10.1038/jid.2012.111.
27. Park SY, Kim HS, Lee SH, et al. Characterization and analysis of the skin microbiota in acne: impact of systemic antibiotics. J Clin Med 2020;9(1):168. https://doi.org/10.3390/jcm9010168.
28. Elvers KT, Wilson VJ, Hammond A, et al. Antibiotic-induced changes in the human gut microbiota for the most commonly prescribed antibiotics in primary care in the UK: a systematic review. BMJ Open 2020;10(9):e035677. https://doi.org/10.1136/bmjopen-2019-035677.

29. Jung GW, Tse JE, Guiha I, et al. Prospective, randomized, open-label trial comparing the safety, efficacy, and tolerability of an acne treatment regimen with and without a probiotic supplement and minocycline in subjects with mild to moderate acne. J Cutan Med Surg 2013;17(2):114–22. https://doi.org/10.2310/7750.2012.12026.
30. Fabbrocini G, Bertona M, Picazo Ó, et al. Supplementation with Lactobacillus rhamnosus SP1 normalises skin expression of genes implicated in insulin signalling and improves adult acne. Benef Microbes 2016;7(5):625–30. https://doi.org/10.3920/BM2016.0089.
31. Paller AS, Mancini AJ. Hurwitz clinical pediatric dermatology: a Textbook of skin disorders of childhood and adolescence. 5th edition. Elsevier; 2016. Available at: **https://www.elsevier.com/books/hurwitz-clinical-pediatric-dermatology/paller/978-0-323-24475-6**. March 13, 2021.
32. Christensen T, Yang JS, Castelo-Soccio L. Bullying and quality of life in pediatric alopecia areata. Skin Appendage Disord 2017;3(3):115–8. https://doi.org/10.1159/000466704.
33. Toussi A, Barton VR, Le ST, et al. Psychosocial and psychiatric comorbidities and health-related quality of life in alopecia areata: a systematic review. J Am Acad Dermatol 2020. https://doi.org/10.1016/j.jaad.2020.06.047.
34. Wang E, Mcelwee KJ. Etiopathogenesis of alopecia areata: why do our patients get it? Dermatol Ther 2011;24(3):337–47. https://doi.org/10.1111/j.1529-8019.2011.01416.x.
35. Kang H, Wu WY, Lo BKK, et al. Hair follicles from alopecia areata patients exhibit alterations in immune privilege-associated gene expression in advance of hair loss. J Invest Dermatol 2010;130(11):2677–80. https://doi.org/10.1038/jid.2010.180.
36. Pinto D, Sorbellini E, Marzani B, et al. Scalp bacterial shift in Alopecia areata. PLoS One 2019;14(4):e0215206. https://doi.org/10.1371/journal.pone.0215206.
37. Moreno-Arrones OM, Serrano-Villar S, Perez-Brocal V, et al. Analysis of the gut microbiota in alopecia areata: identification of bacterial biomarkers. J Eur Acad Dermatol Venereol 2020;34(2):400–5. https://doi.org/10.1111/jdv.15885.
38. Costello ME, Ciccia F, Willner D, et al. Brief report: intestinal dysbiosis in ankylosing spondylitis. Arthritis Rheumatol 2015;67(3):686–91. https://doi.org/10.1002/art.38967.
39. Furusawa Y, Obata Y, Fukuda S, et al. Commensal microbe-derived butyrate induces the differentiation of colonic regulatory T cells. Nature 2013;504(7480):446–50. https://doi.org/10.1038/nature12721.
40. Thompson JM, Mirza MA, Park MK, et al. The role of micronutrients in alopecia areata: a review. Am J Clin Dermatol 2017;18(5):663–79. https://doi.org/10.1007/s40257-017-0285-x.
41. Rebello D, Wang E, Yen E, et al. Hair growth in two alopecia patients after fecal microbiota transplant. ACG Case Rep J 2017;4:e107. https://doi.org/10.14309/crj.2017.107.
42. Kay J, Gawkrodger DJ, Mortimer MJ, et al. The prevalence of childhood atopic eczema in a general population. J Am Acad Dermatol 1994;30(1):35–9. https://doi.org/10.1016/S0190-9622(94)70004-4.
43. Cheng BT, Silverberg JI. Association of pediatric atopic dermatitis and psoriasis with school absenteeism and parental work absenteeism: a cross-sectional United States population-based study. J Am Acad Dermatol 2021. https://doi.org/10.1016/j.jaad.2021.02.069.
44. Daud LR, Garralda ME, David TJ. Psychosocial adjustment in preschool children with atopic eczema. Arch Dis Child 1993;69(6):670–6. https://doi.org/10.1136/adc.69.6.670.
45. Bender BG, Leung SB, Leung DYM. Actigraphy assessment of sleep disturbance in patients with atopic dermatitis: an objective life quality measure. J Allergy Clin Immunol 2003;111(3):598–602. https://doi.org/10.1067/mai.2003.174.
46. Paller AS, Spergel JM, Mina-Osorio P, et al. The atopic march and atopic multimorbidity: many trajectories, many pathways. J Allergy Clin Immunol 2019;143(1):46–55. https://doi.org/10.1016/j.jaci.2018.11.006.
47. Kennedy EA, Connolly J, Hourihane JO, et al. Skin microbiome before development of atopic dermatitis: early colonization with commensal staphylococci at 2 months is associated with a lower risk of atopic dermatitis at 1 year. J Allergy Clin Immunol 2017;139(1):166–72. https://doi.org/10.1016/j.jaci.2016.07.029.
48. Meylan P, Lang C, Mermoud S, et al. Skin colonization by staphylococcus aureus precedes the clinical diagnosis of atopic dermatitis in infancy. J Invest Dermatol 2017;137(12):2497–504. https://doi.org/10.1016/j.jid.2017.07.834.
49. Geoghegan JA, Irvine AD, Foster TJ. Staphylococcus aureus and atopic dermatitis: a complex and evolving relationship. Trends Microbiol 2018;26(6):484–97. https://doi.org/10.1016/j.tim.2017.11.008.
50. Kobayashi T, Glatz M, Horiuchi K, et al. Dysbiosis and staphylococcus aureus colonization drives inflammation in atopic dermatitis. Immunity 2015;42(4):756–66. https://doi.org/10.1016/j.immuni.2015.03.014.
51. Shi B, Bangayan NJ, Curd E, et al. The skin microbiome is different in pediatric versus adult atopic dermatitis. J Allergy Clin Immunol 2016;138(4):1233–6. https://doi.org/10.1016/j.jaci.2016.04.053.

52. Gonzalez ME, Schaffer JV, Orlow SJ, et al. Cutaneous microbiome effects of fluticasone propionate cream and adjunctive bleach baths in childhood atopic dermatitis. J Am Acad Dermatol 2016;75(3): 481–93.e8. https://doi.org/10.1016/j.jaad.2016.04.066.
53. Seite S, Flores GE, Henley JB, et al. Microbiome of affected and unaffected skin of patients with atopic dermatitis before and after emollient treatment. J Drugs Dermatol 2014;13(11):1365–72.
54. Totté JEE, Feltz WT, Hennekam M, et al. Prevalence and odds of Staphylococcus aureus carriage in atopic dermatitis: a systematic review and meta-analysis. Br J Dermatol 2016;175(4):687–95. https://doi.org/10.1111/bjd.14566.
55. Simpson EL, Villarreal M, Jepson B, et al. Patients with atopic dermatitis colonized with staphylococcus aureus have a distinct phenotype and endotype. J Invest Dermatol 2018;138(10):2224–33. https://doi.org/10.1016/j.jid.2018.03.1517.
56. Byrd AL, Deming C, Cassidy SKB, et al. Staphylococcus aureus and Staphylococcus epidermidis strain diversity underlying pediatric atopic dermatitis. Sci Transl Med 2017;9(397):eaal4651. https://doi.org/10.1126/scitranslmed.aal4651.
57. Kong HH, Oh J, Deming C, et al. Temporal shifts in the skin microbiome associated with disease flares and treatment in children with atopic dermatitis. Genome Res 2012;22(5):850–9. https://doi.org/10.1101/gr.131029.111.
58. Guzik TJ, Bzowska M, Kasprowicz A, et al. Persistent skin colonization with Staphylococcus aureus in atopic dermatitis: relationship to clinical and immunological parameters. Clin Exp Allergy 2005; 35(4):448–55. https://doi.org/10.1111/j.1365-2222.2005.02210.x.
59. D'Elios S, Trambusti I, Verduci E, et al. Probiotics in the prevention and treatment of atopic dermatitis. Pediatr Allergy Immunol 2020;31(S26):43–5. https://doi.org/10.1111/pai.13364.
60. Huang R, Ning H, Shen M, et al. Probiotics for the treatment of atopic dermatitis in children: a systematic review and meta-analysis of randomized controlled trials. Front Cell Infect Microbiol 2017;7: 392. https://doi.org/10.3389/fcimb.2017.00392.
61. Zhao M, Shen C, Ma L. Treatment efficacy of probiotics on atopic dermatitis, zooming in on infants: a systematic review and meta-analysis. Int J Dermatol 2018;57(6):635–41. https://doi.org/10.1111/ijd.13873.
62. Nestle FO, Kaplan DH, Barker J. Psoriasis. N Engl J Med 2009;361(5):496–509. https://doi.org/10.1056/NEJMra0804595.
63. Mercy K, Kwasny M, Cordoro KM, et al. Clinical manifestations of pediatric psoriasis: results of a multicenter study in the United States. Pediatr Dermatol 2013;30(4):424–8. https://doi.org/10.1111/pde.12072.
64. Honig PJ. Guttate psoriasis associated with perianal streptococcal disease. J Pediatr 1988;113(6): 1037–9. https://doi.org/10.1016/s0022-3476(88)80577-8.
65. Raychaudhuri SP, Gross J. A comparative study of pediatric onset psoriasis with adult onset psoriasis. Pediatr Dermatol 2000;17(3):174–8. https://doi.org/10.1046/j.1525-1470.2000.01746.x.
66. Leung DY, Travers JB, Giorno R, et al. Evidence for a streptococcal superantigen-driven process in acute guttate psoriasis. J Clin Invest 1995;96(5):2106–12. https://doi.org/10.1172/JCI118263.
67. Valdimarsson H, Baker BS, Jónsdóttir I, et al. Psoriasis: a T-cell-mediated autoimmune disease induced by streptococcal superantigens? Immunol Today 1995;16(3):145–9. https://doi.org/10.1016/0167-5699(95)80132-4.
68. Myers B, Brownstone N, Reddy V, et al. The gut microbiome in psoriasis and psoriatic arthritis. Best Pract Res Clin Rheumatol 2019;33(6):101494. https://doi.org/10.1016/j.berh.2020.101494.
69. Waldman A, Gilhar A, Duek L, et al. Incidence of Candida in psoriasis – a study on the fungal flora of psoriatic patients. Mycoses 2001;44(3–4):77–81. https://doi.org/10.1046/j.1439-0507.2001.00608.x.
70. Lee FI, Bellary SV, Francis C. Increased occurrence of psoriasis in patients with Crohn's disease and their relatives. Am J Gastroenterol 1990;85(8): 962–3.
71. Preus HR, Khanifam P, Kolltveit K, et al. Periodontitis in psoriasis patients: a blinded, case-controlled study. Acta Odontol Scand 2010;68(3):165–70. https://doi.org/10.3109/00016350903583678.
72. Zákostelská Z, Málková J, Klimešová K, et al. Intestinal microbiota promotes psoriasis-like skin inflammation by enhancing Th17 response. PLoS One 2016;11(7):e0159539. https://doi.org/10.1371/journal.pone.0159539.
73. Yeh NL, Hsu CY, Tsai TF, et al. Gut microbiome in psoriasis is perturbed differently during secukinumab and ustekinumab therapy and associated with response to treatment. Clin Drug Investig 2019; 39(12):1195–203. https://doi.org/10.1007/s40261-019-00849-7.
74. Fahlén A, Engstrand L, Baker BS, et al. Comparison of bacterial microbiota in skin biopsies from normal and psoriatic skin. Arch Dermatol Res 2012;304(1): 15–22. https://doi.org/10.1007/s00403-011-1189-x.
75. Chang HW, Yan D, Singh R, et al. Alteration of the cutaneous microbiome in psoriasis and potential role in Th17 polarization. Microbiome 2018;6(1): 154. https://doi.org/10.1186/s40168-018-0533-1.
76. Marples RR, Heaton CL, Kligman AM. Staphylococcus aureus in Psoriasis. Arch Dermatol 1973;

107(4):568–70. https://doi.org/10.1001/archderm.1973.01620190044010.
77. Balci DD, Duran N, Ozer B, et al. High prevalence of Staphylococcus aureus cultivation and superantigen production in patients with psoriasis. Eur J Dermatol 2009;19(3):238–42. https://doi.org/10.1684/ejd.2009.0663.
78. Tomi NS, Kränke B, Aberer E. Staphylococcal toxins in patients with psoriasis, atopic dermatitis, and erythroderma, and in healthy control subjects. J Am Acad Dermatol 2005;53(1):67–72. https://doi.org/10.1016/j.jaad.2005.02.034.
79. Fry L, Baker BS, Powles AV, et al. Is chronic plaque psoriasis triggered by microbiota in the skin? Br J Dermatol 2013;169(1):47–52. https://doi.org/10.1111/bjd.12322.
80. Chen YJ, Ho HJ, Wu CY, et al. Infantile infection and antibiotic exposure in association with pediatric psoriasis development: a nationwide nested case-control study. J Am Acad Dermatol 2020. https://doi.org/10.1016/j.jaad.2020.12.014.
81. Horton DB, Scott FI, Haynes K, et al. Antibiotic exposure, infection, and the development of pediatric psoriasis: a nested case-control study. JAMA Dermatol 2016;152(2):191–9. https://doi.org/10.1001/jamadermatol.2015.3650.
82. Zanvit P, Konkel JE, Jiao X, et al. Antibiotics in neonatal life increase murine susceptibility to experimental psoriasis. Nat Commun 2015;6:8424. https://doi.org/10.1038/ncomms9424.
83. Moises-Alfaro CB, Caceres-Rios HW, Rueda M, et al. Are infantile seborrheic and atopic dermatitis clinical variants of the same disease? Int J Dermatol 2002;41(6):349–51. https://doi.org/10.1046/j.1365-4362.2002.01497.x.
84. Wang L, Clavaud C, Bar-Hen A, et al. Characterization of the major bacterial-fungal populations colonizing dandruff scalps in Shanghai, China, shows microbial disequilibrium. Exp Dermatol 2015;24(5):398–400. https://doi.org/10.1111/exd.12684.
85. Clavaud C, Jourdain R, Bar-Hen A, et al. Dandruff is associated with disequilibrium in the proportion of the major bacterial and fungal populations colonizing the scalp. PLoS One 2013;8(3):e58203. https://doi.org/10.1371/journal.pone.0058203.
86. Xu Z, Wang Z, Yuan C, et al. Dandruff is associated with the conjoined interactions between host and microorganisms. Sci Rep 2016;6:24877. https://doi.org/10.1038/srep24877.
87. Broberg A, Faergemann J. Infantile seborrhoeic dermatitis and Pityrosporum ovale. Br J Dermatol 1989;120(3):359–62. https://doi.org/10.1111/j.1365-2133.1989.tb04160.x.
88. Ruiz-Maldonado R, López-Matínez R, Pérez Chavarría EL, et al. Pityrosporum ovale in infantile seborrheic dermatitis. Pediatr Dermatol 1989;6(1):16–20. https://doi.org/10.1111/j.1525-1470.1989.tb00260.x.
89. Gupta AK, Batra R, Bluhm R, et al. Skin diseases associated with Malassezia species. J Am Acad Dermatol 2004;51(5):785–98. https://doi.org/10.1016/j.jaad.2003.12.034.
90. Pierard GE, Arrese JE, Pierard-Franchimont C, et al. Prolonged effects of antidandruff shampoos - time to recurrence of Malassezia ovalis colonization of skin. Int J Cosmet Sci 1997;19(3):111–7. https://doi.org/10.1046/j.1467-2494.1997.171706.x.
91. Shuster S. The aetiology of dandruff and the mode of action of therapeutic agents. Br J Dermatol 1984;111(2):235–42. https://doi.org/10.1111/j.1365-2133.1984.tb04050.x.
92. Wikramanayake TC, Borda LJ, Miteva M, et al. Seborrheic dermatitis-looking beyond Malassezia. Exp Dermatol 2019;28(9):991–1001. https://doi.org/10.1111/exd.14006.
93. Gaitanis G, Magiatis P, Hantschke M, et al. The Malassezia genus in skin and systemic diseases. Clin Microbiol Rev 2012;25(1):106–41. https://doi.org/10.1128/CMR.00021-11.
94. Ro BI, Dawson TL. The role of sebaceous gland activity and scalp microfloral metabolism in the etiology of seborrheic dermatitis and dandruff. J Investig Dermatol Symp Proc 2005;10(3):194–7. https://doi.org/10.1111/j.1087-0024.2005.10104.x.
95. Henderson CA, Taylor J, Cunliffe WJ. Sebum excretion rates in mothers and neonates. Br J Dermatol 2000;142(1):110–1. https://doi.org/10.1046/j.1365-2133.2000.03249.x.

Systemic Therapy for Vascular Anomalies and the Emergence of Genotype-Guided Management

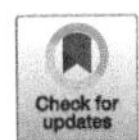

Cynthia L. Nicholson, MD[a], Sheilagh M. Maguiness, MD[b,*]

KEYWORDS

• Vascular malformations • Genetic mutations • Medical management • Emerging therapies

KEY POINTS

- The genetic basis for several vascular anomalies has been elucidated.
- The genetic mutations responsible for the development of vascular anomalies may serve as therapeutic targets for challenging lesions.
- Selective inhibition of MEK, Ras, AKT, PIK3CA, and mTOR is among the most commonly reported targets in the treatment of vascular anomalies.
- Medical management of vascular anomalies is an emerging field in which numerous studies are currently underway.

INTRODUCTION

Vascular anomalies are estimated to affect between 4% and 5% of individuals.[1] In 1996, the International Society for the Study of Vascular Anomalies (ISSVA) recognized the need to classify vascular lesions and proposed a broad division between tumors and malformations. Vascular tumors harbor a potential for proliferation, whereas malformations were generally thought to be related to errors in vasculogenesis.[2] Since this initial binary classification system, more vascular anomalies, along with the genetic basis for their development, have been characterized leading to updates within the ISSVA classification system. Improved understanding of the genetic basis for numerous vascular anomalies has laid the foundation for the emergence of targeted medical therapies as viable treatment options.

The diagnosis of vascular anomalies can present a significant challenge owing to overlapping features and heterogeneity in presentation. Vascular tumors are classified as benign, locally aggressive, or borderline lesions. In contrast, vascular malformations are divided into a more complex system with simple, combined vascular malformations, anomalies of major named vessels, and those associated with other anomalies/syndromes.[3] Many vascular anomalies are relatively uncomplicated and do not require intervention. However, other complex lesions may be complicated by hematologic, cardiac, pulmonary, or neurologic compromise, and in some cases, there is a risk for mortality. There is a need for therapeutic options when vascular anomalies cannot be managed with either interventional radiologic techniques or surgical resection. With improved knowledge of the genetic cause of many vascular anomalies, the concept of tailored, genetically targeted management is an actively emerging field.

[a] Division of Pediatric Dermatology, Department of Dermatology, University of Minnesota, 2512 South Seventh Street, Floor 3, Minneapolis, MN, USA; [b] Division of Pediatric Dermatology, Department of Dermatology, University of Minnesota, 2512 S 7th st, Minneapolis, MN 55454, USA
* Corresponding author.
E-mail address: smaguine@umn.edu

Dermatol Clin 40 (2022) 127–136
https://doi.org/10.1016/j.det.2021.12.009
0733-8635/22/© 2022 Elsevier Inc. All rights reserved.

DISCUSSION

Key Molecular Pathways (VEGF, Ras/Raf/MEK/ERK, PI3K/AKT/mTOR)

Several distinct molecular pathways are well established in the oncology literature. Mutations in proteins within these pathways are directly linked to cancer formation or predisposition. Several of these pathways are shared with overgrowth syndromes. As knowledge of the genetic basis of vascular anomalies has increased with time, mutations within these same molecular pathways have been identified as relevant contributors to the pathogenesis of vascular anomalies.[4] Each pathway harbors potential therapeutic targets (**Fig. 1**).

Vascular endothelial growth factor (VEGF) is intricately tied to all vasculogenesis, angiogenesis, and the development of lymphatic vessels. Signal transduction occurs via binding to receptor tyrosine kinases. Primary congenital lymphedema, Meige disease, and hypotrichosis lymphedema telangiectasia are some of the conditions genetically related to signal transduction errors within this pathway.[4]

Ras/Raf/MEK/ERK is critically important in endothelial cell function, and faulty signaling at any step within this pathway can lead to the development of vascular anomalies.[4] This pathway is among the most well-described pathways implicated in the pathogenesis of vascular anomalies. Beyond its role in vasculogenesis, mutations in this pathway are well known in oncology, as mutations in these genes result in numerous cancers and cancer predisposition syndromes.[5] Ras is a small GTP-binding protein that is responsible for activating Raf. Four different Ras protein variants have been identified and show variable propensity to activate the subsequent steps in signal transmission.[5,6] Farnesylation in combination with other posttranslational modifications allows Ras to subsequently target the cell membrane.[6] In coordination with cytokines, growth factors, and mitogens, Ras is activated after exchange of GDP for GTP, which then activates Raf.[7,8] Raf, a serine/threonine kinase, is activated by a complicated interaction between dimerization, phosphorylation, or dephosphorylation of regulatory sites and dissociation from regularly proteins.[5,7] Raf activation results in activation of mitogen-activated protein kinase/ERK kinase (MEK1).[5] MEK1 is a protein kinase that primarily targets activation by phosphorylation of ERK. This pathway is vitally important in cell growth, malignancy, transformation, and even aging.[9] Of note, Ras is a common upstream regulator to other pathways, including PI3K/protein kinase B (AKT), for which there are existing therapeutic targets.[7,9] Ras variants differ in their ability to activate both the Ras/Raf/MEK/ERK pathway and the PI3K pathway.[5]

Dysregulation of the PI3K/AKT/mTOR pathway is another relevant player in the development of vascular anomalies and in basic cellular function, including proliferation, migration, metabolic function, and viability.[4] Anomalous activation of this pathway is similarly implicated in metabolic disorders and malignancy.[9] Similar mechanisms, that is, loss of function of phosphatase and tensin homolog (PTEN), which functions as a negative regulator of this pathway, Ras mutations, or dysregulated expression of growth factors, leads to the development of both cancer and vascular malformations.[4,10] Signal transduction within this pathway occurs through an important interaction between the alpha subunit of PI3K, p110α, and is responsible for the conversion of phosphatidylinositol (3,4) biphosphate (PIP2) into phosphatidylinositol (3,4,5)-triphosphate (PIP3).[11] Subsequent activation of 3-phosphoinositide-dependent-kinase-1 and phosphorylation of AKT allow for activation of the rapamycin complex 1 (mTORc1).[11]

The remaining 2 pathways, transforming growth factor-β (TGF-β) and angiopoietin-TIE-2 pathways, are also involved in endothelial cell function and implicated in the pathogenesis of certain vascular malformations.

Lymphatic Malformations

Lymphatic malformations are slow-flow vascular lesions related to abnormal development of the lymphatic system.[12] Although lymphatic malformations can be found in nearly any region of the body, they most frequently are identified in lymphatic-rich regions.[13] Approximately 48% are found in the head and neck region, whereas 42% are found in the trunk and extremities.[14] Lymphatic malformations occur between 1.2 and 2.8 per 1000 births.[15]

Lymphatic vessels are lined by a single-layer endothelium and are filled with proteinaceous material, but red blood cells commonly seen as spontaneous hemorrhage are not uncommon.[13] The distinction between microcystic and macrocystic lymphatic anomalies is determined by the size of the cyst, with those less than 1 cm classified as microcystic, whereas those larger than 1 cm are classified as macrocystic.[16] Ultrasound is a relatively inexpensive and widely available imaging technique used to visualize lymphatic anomalies, but if further details are required for diagnosis or characterization, MRI can be obtained.

Lymphatic malformations are generally sporadic but can occur in the setting of genetic syndromes. The most frequently identified mutation in

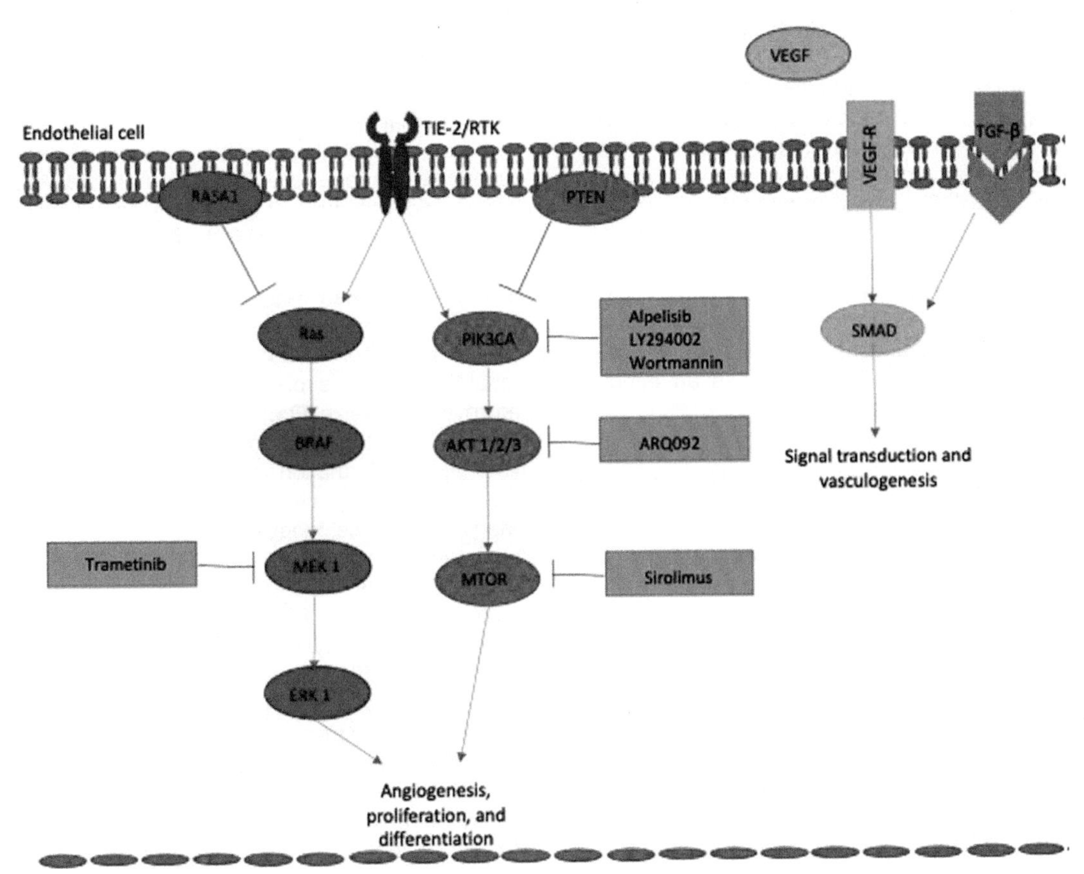

Fig. 1. Five key pathways implicated in the development of vascular anomalies are outlined in this figure. Interruption or uninhibited signaling at any of the critical steps can lead to the development of a vascular anomaly. Targetable checkpoints by medical management with alpelisib, trametinib, sirolimus, and others can interrupt uninhibited signaling.

lymphatic malformations found in the head and neck region is in the PIK3CA-related gene.[17,18]

Although macrocystic lymphatic malformations may be managed with surgical excision or sclerotherapy, the invasive and infiltrative nature of microcysts and mixed macro/microcystic lesions often presents a therapeutic challenge.[19,20] Identification of somatic mutations in lymphatic malformations has allowed targeted therapies to play a role in the management of these previously inoperable and potentially devastating malformations.

Kaposiform Hemangioendothelioma

Kaposiform hemangioendothelioma (KHE) is a rare vascular tumor occurring with an incidence of approximately 0.071 per 100,000 children.[21] KHE can have a variable presentation as a nodule or mass with prominent overlying purpuric vasculature.[22] However, KHEs may also have a more infiltrative appearance that is ill defined, occupying a broader region. The lateral neck, axilla, groin, extremities, and trunk are most commonly affected, but noncutaneous involvement has also been reported.[23] Unfortunately, because of a varied presentation, its association with Kasabach-Merritt phenomenon (KMP), and no standardized treatment approaches, this rare vascular tumor is associated with significant morbidity and mortality.

It is hypothesized that disrupted angiogenesis and lymphangiogenesis lead to the development of KHE. However, this process is yet to be clearly defined. Expression via the VEGF-C and VEGF receptor 3 pathway is important in lymphatic growth and also is found highly expressed in KHEs, likely contributing to their aggressive and infiltrative behavior.[22] Angiopoietin-2 (Ang-2) is also found to be elevated in patients with KHE. Signaling through the angiopoietin pathway is important during vessel development and lymphangiogenesis. Ang-2 signaling through TIE-2 activates the AKT/mTOR pathway and likely explains the efficacy of sirolimus in KHE management.[22] More recently, few reports of KHE and tufted angioma were found to have somatic mutations in GNA14, thus highlighting a potential role in MAPK inhibition.[24,25]

Platelet trapping and a subsequent consumptive coagulopathy can complicate a KHE. This clinically presents with a sudden increase in size of the tumor, and this phenomenon is known as KMP. Elevated D-dimer, fibrin degradation products, hypofibrinogenemia, and thrombocytopenia are seen in KMP. This phenomenon is life-threatening and puts patients at high risk for hemorrhage. Surgical interventions are only recommended in extreme circumstances, as invasive procedures can worsen a coagulopathy or trigger the cascade in situations where it is not yet active. However, it has been reported as an effective modality in limited cases.[26]

Sirolimus: A Promising Medical Therapy for Lymphatic Malformations and Kaposiform Hemangioendothelioma

Sirolimus is one of the first systemic therapies with reported evidence for the treatment of lymphatic malformations and KHE. Sirolimus is a macrolide derived from *Streptomyces hygroscopicus* and inhibits mTOR, thus halting downstream signal transduction in the PI3K/AKT/mTOR pathway.[17] The most frequent use is for prevention of post-transplant rejection.[17]

In 2011, one of the first reports of oral sirolimus in vascular anomalies was published.[27] Six patients were granted compassionate use for treatment. Four of these patients had a lymphatic microcystic malformation, one with a capillary lymphatic-venous malformation, and the last one was diagnosed with KHE, which was complicated by KMP. All 6 patients experienced a dramatic response to sirolimus. Normalization of coagulation parameters, improvement in cardiac function, and respiratory status were achieved.[27] This landmark article set the stage for a dramatic shift in management for previously untreatable vascular anomalies and supported a research initiative to grow knowledge of medical management for vascular anomalies.

Safety data gleaned from studies on vascular anomalies support its use as a safe and efficacious treatment option.[28] In a systematic review article by Freixo and colleagues,[29] 73 articles were reviewed in which 317 patients were treated with oral sirolimus for a vascular anomaly. Oral mucositis was the most common side effect, which occurred in 31.9% of patients, dyslipidemia occurred in 16.5%, leukopenia occurred in 12.3%, gastrointestinal symptoms occurred in 10.2%, and rash occurred in 8.2%.

Efficacy data have slowly emerged in the literature, but one of the major contributors is from a large systematic review reported by Wiegand and colleagues,[15] who reviewed the treatment of lymphatic malformations in 71 patients who received sirolimus. Sixty of those patients experienced partial remission; only 3 had progression or a lack of response, and the outcome of 8 patients was not reported. Airway compromise is a feared and potentially devastating complication of lymphatic malformations in the neck region. Historically, Lymphatic Malformations (LMs) in this location have been treated by surgical intervention, but prior studies demonstrate that this can be avoided in some cases.[30] In the authors' personal experience, sirolimus can lead to dramatic improvement in size. **Fig. 2** demonstrates a patient with an extensive microcystic and macrocystic lymphatic malformation involving the face, neck, submandibular space, sublingual space, retropharyngeal space, deep neck soft tissues, and left anterior chest wall with improvement in volume on oral sirolimus (see **Fig. 2**).

With respect to KHE, the rarity of this tumor precludes the ability to perform randomized controlled trials to assess efficacy of various treatment modalities. Rather, expert recommendations and personal experience guide management decisions. Based on consensus guidelines, vincristine with or without corticosteroids is recommended for the treatment of KHE complicated by KMP.[23] However, since 2010, reports of sirolimus have emerged in the literature.[27] In a retrospective review of 26 patients treated with sirolimus for KHE, 25 of which were also complicated by KMP, for a duration of 28.3 ± 12.5 months, 19 of them reduced to small residual lesions. The average time to response was about 1 week with few reported side effects.[31] In another retrospective study involving 52 patients with progressive KHE that were treated with sirolimus, significant decreases in severity of the tumors were noted at 6 and 12 months.[32] Of this cohort, 37 patients exhibited KMP, whereas the remainder did not, and the response to treatment was more pronounced in those who had KMP.[32] Although vincristine is considered to be a first-line treatment in patients with KHE complicated by KMP, the ease of administration of sirolimus in combination with the safety profile makes it a reasonable first choice. In the authors' opinion, treatment endpoint of sirolimus for KHE is complicated, as recurrence or progression of the tumor is expected with discontinuation. In prior cases, treatment endpoint has been dictated by symptom management, in combination with normalization of coagulation parameters and size. However, in most cases, long-term treatment, intermittent treatment, or adjunctive therapies, such as surgical intervention, will be needed. Vincristine has been compared

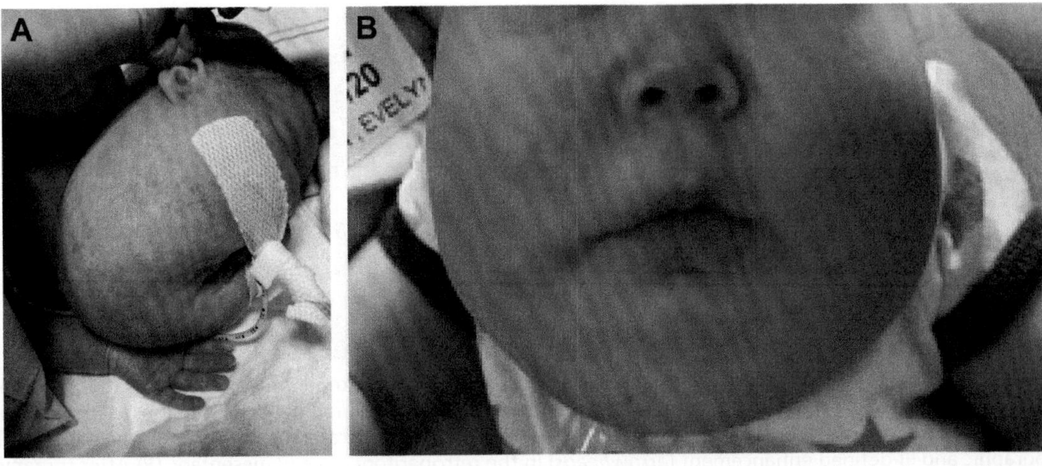

Fig. 2. (*A*) A large microcystic and macrocystic lymphatic malformation is observed at birth. Oral sirolimus was started shortly after delivery. (*B*) A dramatic improvement in the volume of the malformation can be observed at 4 months of life.

with sirolimus in a meta-analysis of 15 studies performed in 2019 of KHE with or without KMP, which supported its use as an initial agent when compared with vincristine.[33]

In the authors' experience with KHE complicated by KMP, sirolimus monotherapy has been successful in treating a complicated multifocal KHE, including a mediastinal mass that presented with retroperitoneal hemorrhage with a platelet nadir of 21 $\times$ 10^9 per liter. In **Fig. 3**A, portions of the vascular tumor invading the retroperitoneal space at presentation can be seen, and improvement after treatment with sirolimus can be seen in **Fig. 3**B. This child remains on therapy at 12 months of age and was started at 2 months when he presented with active platelet consumption. Sirolimus was also effective in another recent case at the authors' institution of a KHE located in the occipital scalp that presented with a lower-grade consumptive coagulopathy at 7 weeks of age (**Fig. 4**A). This patient remains stable on treatment at 18 months of age without any serious adverse side effects (**Fig. 4**B). Discussions regarding definitive surgical resection are underway but are complicated by a somewhat broad residual tumor base.

Varying dosing regimens for sirolimus have been suggested. The standard dosing among many articles is an initial dose of 0.8 mg/m^2 per dose twice daily with titration based on target blood levels, which usually range between 4 and 15 ng/mL.[15] Studies published after this review and from personal experience have generally aligned with the above recommendations.

Some limitations to standardizing the use of sirolimus in complicated and inoperable microcystic lymphatic malformations and in KHE are related to a paucity of randomized controlled trials available to objectively assess improvement. Most of the data are obtained from limited case series that report improvement based on subjective findings. However, studies are ongoing in the pediatric population with an effort to create evidence-based guidelines, which will lend to evidence-based decision making.[34]

PIK3CA-Related Overgrowth Syndromes

Mutations in the PIK3CA gene have been found in several known overgrowth syndromes. Growth is largely regulated by this gene. When postzygotic or somatic mutations in this gene occur, varying presentations develop depending on when the mutation occurs in embryogenesis. Although isolated macrodactyly can develop in a late somatic mutation in this gene, more severe presentations occur if a disruption occurs earlier in development. With significant phenotypic variation in presentation, this has led to the relatively recent reclassification of these overgrowth syndromes based on their genetic basis, termed the PIK3CA Overgrowth Syndromes (PROS). This heterogeneous group of disorders includes congenital lipomatous, overgrowth, vascular malformations, epidermal nevi and scoliosis/skeletal/spinal anomalies (CLOVES syndrome), macrodactyly and muscle hemihypertrophy, megalencephaly-capillary malformation (MCM) and hemimegalencephaly, fibroadipose hyperplasia or overgrowth, dysplastic megalencephaly, and Klippel Trenaunay (KT) syndrome.[35] These diseases are characterized by asymmetric overgrowth in combination with vascular anomalies, neurologic findings, and changes to the internal organ systems.[36] Although

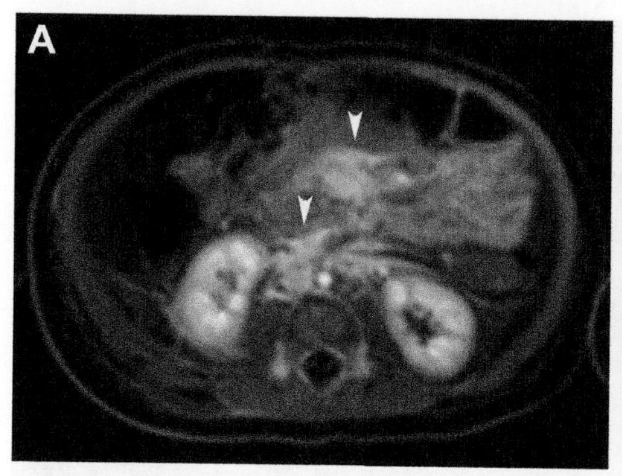

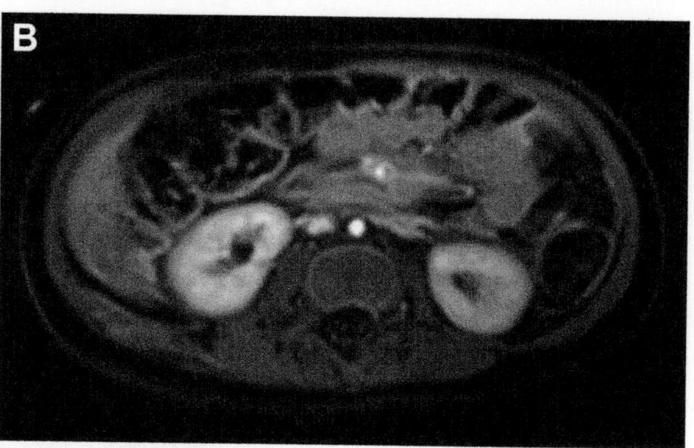

Fig. 3. (*A*) Before therapy: postcontrast axial T1-weighted image in the arterial phase and with fat saturation. Multicentric KHE lesion in a 3-month-old male infant. Although there were more superficial lesions in the extremity that were not visualized on MRI, the intra-abdominal lesions were transspatial and infiltrative. There is geographic and ill-defined enhancement (*arrowheads*) in the retroperitoneum and mesentery. (*B*) After therapy: postcontrast axial T1-weighted image in the arterial phase and with fat saturation. The transspatial and infiltrative enhancing lesions noted on panel A have markedly improved after medical therapy. There is no substantial residual enhancement within the affected area, and through the remainder of the examination, only a trace amount of residual abnormal enhancement was noted (not included in the provided image).

there is significant overlap among these conditions, the differential diagnosis remains broad during workup and includes proteus syndrome, PTEN hamartoma syndrome, and neurofibromatosis among others.[35]

Constitutive activation via signaling through MTORc1, as described above, leads to the constellation of findings classically described in PROS.[11] Suggested workup for patients who have findings suspicious for a PROS include imaging of the involved region by MRI, including whole-body MRI if there is truncal involvement, brain MRI for neurologic or facial findings, and spinal imaging in young infants to rule out lipomyelomeningocele.[35] Ongoing surveillance for Wilms tumor with renal ultrasound at baseline and every 3 months until 8 years of age is also suggested because of a documented diagnosis of Wilms tumor in a patient diagnosed with CLOVES syndrome.[35,37]

PIK3CA Overgrowth Syndromes and Systemic Therapies

Historically, treatments for PROS have largely been unsatisfying and limited to surgical debulking and laser interventions for the vascular malformations, but local interventions fail to selectively target the molecular underpinnings responsible for causing the multisystem effects.[36]

Sirolimus

Sirolimus was identified as a viable treatment option for those affected by a PROS. Sirolimus binds

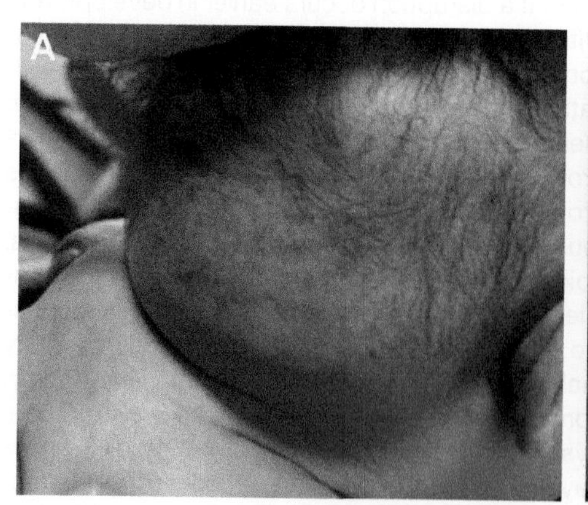

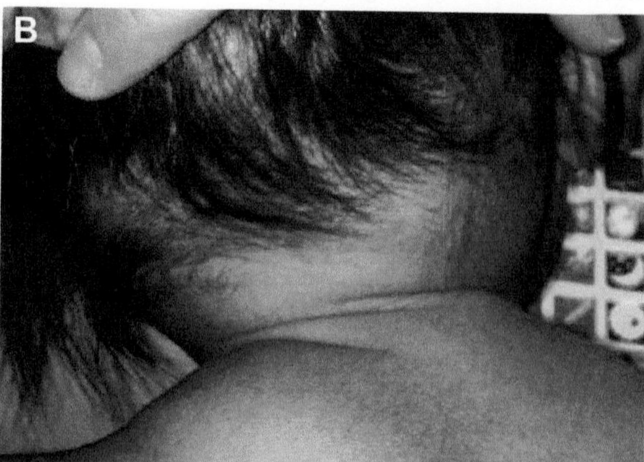

Fig. 4. A large vascular tumor with overlying telangiectasias (*A*) when this patient who was later diagnosed with a KHE presented at 7 weeks of age. The patient remains on oral sirolimus monotherapy with interval improvement noted in follow-up photograph at 17 months of age (*B*).

FKBP12, forming a complex called FKBP12-rapamycin, which binds to mTORc1, thus preventing substrate binding and halting cell-cycle progression.[38] Reported side effects are similar to those described in the transplant and cancer literature and align with those reported in the treatment of lymphatic malformations with sirolimus. Hyperglycemia, stomatitis, pneumonitis, hyperlipidemia, hypertriglyceridemia, bone marrow suppression, and infection are the primary concerns.[35]

Sirolimus was originally reported in CLOVES syndrome in 2 cases that were treated for more than 4 years and 14 months with low-dose sirolimus, which was well tolerated other than hypertriglyceridemia.[36] These findings were corroborated in a larger multicenter trial in which 39 patients with PROS were treated with low-dose sirolimus in a study by Parker and colleagues.[39] Dual-energy X-ray absorptiometry was used as an objective assessment to monitor response. Although efficacy was observed, unfortunately a significant majority of patients experienced adverse effects, but only 7 discontinued treatment.[39]

PIK3CA inhibitors [BYL719 (alpelisib)]

More targeted therapies, including PIK3CA inhibitors, have emerged and may offer more promising results. In 2015, dermal fibroblasts from 3 patients with a PROS were isolated. When sequestered alone, unchecked growth was observed, but in the presence of highly specific PI3K inhibitors, wortmannin and LY294002, their growth potential diminished.[40] These findings were instrumental in the identification of additional agents with therapeutic potential. PI3K, AKT, and mTOR are implicated in the development of cancer, and therefore, these therapeutic targets and research can be reasonably repurposed for this subset of overgrowth disorders.[35]

In the landmark article by Venot and colleagues,[11] BYL719, a highly targeted PIK3CA inhibitor to the alpha fraction, now known as Alpelisib, was approved for compassionate use in 2 patients with life-threatening complications of PROS. Initially, mouse models were used to demonstrate a reduction in tumor volume and showed promising results when compared with the effects of rapamycin. The first patient had numerous complications, including spinal cord compression, heart failure, and kidney disease, whereas the second patient's lymphangioma had extensive involvement of the left kidney and gastrointestinal tract. Traditional therapies were unsuccessful, but after treatment with BYL719, reduced tumor burden, weight loss, and normalization of organ function were observed.[11]

These preliminary results supported broader administration of BYL719 to 17 additional patients with PROS. Patients within this cohort were diagnosed with CLOVES, MCM, and localized overgrowth syndrome. Interestingly, 8 of these patients were recalcitrant to oral sirolimus, but demonstrated improvement in clinical findings and pain control and did not require further surgical intervention.[11] The reported side effects were minimal, which included mouth ulcerations, which spontaneously resolved, transient hyperglycemia, and dose modification of diabetic medications in a previously diabetic patient.[11]

Alpelisib, a highly specific and targeted molecule, is preferrable because of a theoretic reduction in risk of more broad inhibition and is currently being tested in controlled trials as a chemotherapeutic agent.[41] In one early report, a 17-year-old girl formally diagnosed with CLOVES syndrome, complicated by extensive genital vascular malformation, was treated with this agent under compassionate use approval, with resolution of repeated vaginal bleeding and avoidance of further surgical intervention.[41] Alpelisib is a promising therapeutic with significant potential to change the progressive and often devastating course for those affected by a PROS. Clinical trials assessing efficacy of Alpelisib for overgrowth syndromes are ongoing.

Arteriovenous Malformations

Arteriovenous malformations (AVMs) are vascular anomalies in which a direct connection between an artery and a vein exists but lacks an intervening capillary system.[42] These high-flow vascular malformations have a propensity for growth and local destruction and can even lead to death or high-output cardiac failure.[13] The head and neck, extremities, brain, and spinal cord are common locations for AVMs.[43] AVMs are typically congenital, but may stay quiescent during the early years of life and present later during a period of growth.

Most often, AVMs occur as a sporadic finding; in these cases, genetic alterations in MAP2K1 and KRAS have been identified.[42,44,45] However, they can also be syndromic, as seen in capillary malformation-arteriovenous malformation (CM-AVM) syndrome, PTEN hamartoma syndrome, hereditary hemorrhagic telangiectasia (HHT), and CLOVES syndrome.[43] In the case of CM-AVM, PTEN, and HHT, germline mutations in several genes within the Ras/MAPK pathway are well-established causes. Chemotherapeutic agents that target this pathway exist.

Arteriovenous Malformations and Systemic Therapies

Although prior studies had demonstrated that MAP2K1 mutations within endothelial cells were responsible for the development of sporadic AVMs, the translation of this basic science work was demonstrated when signal transduction was blocked in AVM-derived endothelial cells in the presence of Trametinib, a Food and Drug Administration–approved MEK1 inhibitor.[42]

Scattered case reports have since documented use of trametinib for the treatment of AVMs. In 2019, trametinib was used in an 11-year-old girl who was found to have an AVM associated with a MAP2K1 mutation.[46] Sirolimus was used before trametinib, but despite good tolerance, disease control was not achieved.[46] In comparison, trametinib led to clinical improvement after 1 month with the tolerable side effect of an acneiform eruption.[46] KRAS mutations are reported in other AVMs, particularly those involving the central nervous system.[45] Trametinib was used in a KRAS-mutated AVM in the setting of Cobb syndrome. Efficacy was assessed by following improvement in cardiac output and by imaging. The side effects included paronychia, stomatitis, and an acneiform eruption, all of which are reported side effects and did not prevent continued treatment for this patient.[47]

The authors have personal experience in the successful management of a complicated AVM in the setting of CM-AVM syndrome caused by an EPHB4 mutation. The patient's AVM led to cardiac compromise and was not amenable to embolization. This patient is currently being treated with trametinib. Unfortunately, her treatment response is complicated by several side effects, including an acneiform eruption, paronychia, and color changes of the hair, but cardiac function has significantly improved.

Future Directions

The development of additional targeted therapies for management of various vascular anomalies is ongoing. It is reasonable to hypothesize that research done in the oncologic domain will further serve patients with vascular lesions not amenable to standard therapy in the future.

Although a paucity of therapeutics is available that target the TGF-β and angiopoietin-TIE-2 pathways, there is future potential for it to serve as a target. The TGF-β pathway, which signals via serine/threonine kinases, is relevant to both HHT type 1 and 2. TGF-β was recently touted in the literature as a potential therapeutic target in malignancy owing to a diverse interplay between the above-mentioned pathways.[48,49]

ARQ092 is an experimental, oral agent that inhibits AKT.[50] It is under consideration for treatment of cancer, PROS, and proteus syndrome. Initial data from in vitro cell samples cultured from 6 individuals with a PROS demonstrated inhibition of proliferation.[51] When compared with other inhibitors of the PI3K/AKT/mTOR pathway, sirolimus, wortmannin, LY249002, the evidence of cytotoxicity was reduced.[51]

NVP-BEZ235, a dual PI3K and mTOR inhibitor, was also studied in fibroblast cell lines and compared with rapamycin, aspirin, and metformin in the ability to suppress cell growth.[52] Although all agents were able to suppress cell growth, this article suggested that metformin be considered a candidate drug for treating PROS. In this study, metformin did not inhibit control fibroblast cell lines to the same degree as the other agents. The authors suggested that this may be favorable for treatment in the pediatric population when considering the anticipated growth and development in these patients.[52]

SUMMARY

Before 2010, medical management for vascular anomalies was not considered possible. Improved understanding of the genetic underpinnings for both vascular tumors and malformations has put targeted therapeutics within arm's reach. It is likely that in the next decade, genotype-guided therapies will become more commonly used and studied in the field of vascular anomalies. This is an exciting and rapidly evolving area with the potential to significantly benefit patients whose vascular anomalies are not amenable to surgical or interventional radiology-based management.

CLINICS CARE POINTS

- Characterization of vascular anomalies is a rapidly changing field.
- Genetic mutations harbored within vascular anomalies can serve as a therapeutic target for those not amenable to surgical or interventional radiologic techniques.
- Genotype-guided management will become increasingly more accessible for difficult-to-manage vascular anomalies.

ACKNOWLEDGMENTS

The authors would like to thank Michael Murati, MD for his contributions to this article and expertise in radiologic imaging.

DISCLOSURE

Dr S.M. Maguiness has participated in an advisory board for Verrica Pharmaceuticals and has been an investigator for Regeneron Sanofi. She is the co-founder of Stryke Club, a personal care brand for teen boys.

REFERENCES

1. Greene AK. Vascular anomalies: current overview of the field. Clin Plast Surg 2011;38(1):1–5.
2. Wassef M, Blei F, Adams D, et al. Vascular anomalies classification: recommendations from the International Society for the Study of Vascular Anomalies. Pediatrics 2015;136(1):e203–14.
3. ISSVA Classification of Vascular Anomalies ©. Published 2018. Available at: https://www.issva.org/classification. Accessed 02/15/2020.
4. Pang C, Lim CS, Brookes J, et al. Emerging importance of molecular pathogenesis of vascular malformations in clinical practice and classifications. Vasc Med 2020;25(4):364–77.
5. McCubrey JA, Steelman LS, Chappell WH, et al. Roles of the Raf/MEK/ERK pathway in cell growth, malignant transformation and drug resistance. Biochim Biophys Acta 2007;1773(8):1263–84.
6. Chang F, Steelman LS, Lee JT, et al. Signal transduction mediated by the Ras/Raf/MEK/ERK pathway from cytokine receptors to transcription factors: potential targeting for therapeutic intervention. Leukemia 2003;17(7):1263–93.
7. Asati V, Mahapatra DK, Bharti SK. PI3K/Akt/mTOR and Ras/Raf/MEK/ERK signaling pathways inhibitors as anticancer agents: structural and pharmacological perspectives. Eur J Med Chem 2016;109:314–41.
8. McCubrey JA, Steelman LS, Chappell WH, et al. Mutations and deregulation of Ras/Raf/MEK/ERK and PI3K/PTEN/Akt/mTOR cascades which alter therapy response. Oncotarget 2012;3(9):954–87.
9. Chappell WH, Steelman LS, Long JM, et al. Ras/Raf/MEK/ERK and PI3K/PTEN/Akt/mTOR inhibitors: rationale and importance to inhibiting these pathways in human health. Oncotarget 2011;2(3):135–64.
10. Piguet AC, Dufour JF. PI(3)K/PTEN/AKT pathway. J Hepatol 2011;54(6):1317–9.
11. Venot Q, Blanc T, Rabia SH, et al. Targeted therapy in patients with PIK3CA-related overgrowth syndrome. Nature 2018;558(7711):540–6.
12. Elluru RG, Balakrishnan K, Padua HM. Lymphatic malformations: diagnosis and management. Semin Pediatr Surg 2014;23(4):178–85.
13. McCuaig CC. Update on classification and diagnosis of vascular malformations. Curr Opin Pediatr 2017;29(4):448–54.
14. Alqahtani A, Nguyen LT, Flageole H, et al. 25 years' experience with lymphangiomas in children. J Pediatr Surg 1999;34(7):1164–8.
15. Wiegand S, Wichmann G, Dietz A. Treatment of lymphatic malformations with the mTOR inhibitor sirolimus: a systematic review. Lymphat Res Biol 2018;16(4):330–9.
16. Bagrodia N, Defnet AM, Kandel JJ. Management of lymphatic malformations in children. Curr Opin Pediatr 2015;27(3):356–63.
17. Padia R, Zenner K, Bly R, et al. Clinical application of molecular genetics in lymphatic malformations. Laryngoscope Investig Otolaryngol 2019;4(1):170–3.
18. Blesinger H, Kaulfuß S, Aung T, et al. PIK3CA mutations are specifically localized to lymphatic endothelial cells of lymphatic malformations. PLoS One 2018;13(7):e0200343.
19. Bonilla-Velez J, Moore BP, Cleves MA, et al. Surgical resection of macrocystic lymphatic malformations of the head and neck: short and long-term outcomes. Int J Pediatr Otorhinolaryngol 2020;134:110013.
20. Bouwman F, Kooijman SS, Verhoeven BH, et al. Lymphatic malformations in children: treatment outcomes of sclerotherapy in a large cohort. Eur J Pediatr 2021;180(3):959–66.
21. Croteau SE, Liang MG, Kozakewich HP, et al. Kaposiform hemangioendothelioma: atypical features and risks of Kasabach-Merritt phenomenon in 107 referrals. J Pediatr 2013;162(1):142–7.
22. Ji Y, Chen S, Yang K, et al. Kaposiform hemangioendothelioma: current knowledge and future perspectives. Orphanet J Rare Dis 2020;15(1):39.
23. Drolet BA, Trenor CC 3rd, Brandão LR, et al. Consensus-derived practice standards plan for complicated Kaposiform hemangioendothelioma. J Pediatr 2013;163(1):285–91.
24. Lim YH, Bacchiocchi A, Qiu J, et al. GNA14 somatic mutation causes congenital and sporadic vascular tumors by MAPK activation. Am J Hum Genet 2016;99(2):443–50.
25. Lim YH, Fraile C, Antaya RJ, et al. Tufted angioma with associated Kasabach-Merritt phenomenon caused by somatic mutation in GNA14. Pediatr Dermatol 2019;36(6):963–4.
26. Wu Y, Qiu R, Zeng L, et al. Effective surgical treatment of life-threatening huge vascular anomalies associated with thrombocytopenia and coagulopathy in infants unresponsive to drug therapy. BMC Pediatr 2020;20(1):187.

27. Hammill AM, Wentzel M, Gupta A, et al. Sirolimus for the treatment of complicated vascular anomalies in children. Pediatr Blood Cancer 2011;57(6):1018–24.
28. Adams DM, Trenor CC 3rd, Hammill AM, et al. Efficacy and safety of sirolimus in the treatment of complicated vascular anomalies. Pediatrics 2016; 137(2):e20153257.
29. Freixo C, Ferreira V, Martins J, et al. Efficacy and safety of sirolimus in the treatment of vascular anomalies: a systematic review. J Vasc Surg 2020;71(1): 318–27.
30. Triana P, Miguel M, Díaz M, et al. Oral sirolimus: an option in the management of neonates with life-threatening upper airway lymphatic malformations. Lymphat Res Biol 2019;17(5):504–11.
31. Wang Z, Yao W, Sun H, et al. Sirolimus therapy for Kaposiform hemangioendothelioma with long-term follow-up. J Dermatol 2019;46(11):956–61.
32. Ji Y, Chen S, Xiang B, et al. Sirolimus for the treatment of progressive Kaposiform hemangioendothelioma: a multicenter retrospective study. Int J Cancer 2017;141(4):848–55.
33. Peng S, Yang K, Xu Z, et al. Vincristine and sirolimus in the treatment of Kaposiform haemangioendothelioma. J Paediatr Child Health 2019;55(9):1119–24.
34. Maruani A, Boccara O, Bessis D, et al. Treatment of voluminous and complicated superficial slow-flow vascular malformations with sirolimus (PERFORMUS): protocol for a multicenter phase 2 trial with a randomized observational-phase design. Trials 2018;19(1):340.
35. Keppler-Noreuil KM, Rios JJ, Parker VE, et al. PIK3CA-related overgrowth spectrum (PROS): diagnostic and testing eligibility criteria, differential diagnosis, and evaluation. Am J Med Genet A 2015; 167a(2):287–95.
36. Martinez-Lopez A, Blasco-Morente G, Perez-Lopez I, et al. CLOVES syndrome: review of a PIK3CA-related overgrowth spectrum (PROS). Clin Genet 2017;91(1):14–21.
37. Kurek KC, Luks VL, Ayturk UM, et al. Somatic mosaic activating mutations in PIK3CA cause CLOVES syndrome. Am J Hum Genet 2012;90(6): 1108–15.
38. Sehgal SN. Sirolimus: its discovery, biological properties, and mechanism of action. Transplant Proc 2003;35(3 Suppl):7s–14s.
39. Parker VER, Keppler-Noreuil KM, Faivre L, et al. Safety and efficacy of low-dose sirolimus in the PIK3CA-related overgrowth spectrum. Genet Med 2019;21(5):1189–98.
40. Loconte DC, Grossi V, Bozzao C, et al. Molecular and functional characterization of three different postzygotic mutations in PIK3CA-related overgrowth spectrum (PROS) patients: effects on PI3K/AKT/mTOR signaling and sensitivity to PIK3 inhibitors. PLoS One 2015;10(4):e0123092.
41. López Gutiérrez JC, Lizarraga R, Delgado C, et al. Alpelisib treatment for genital vascular malformation in a patient with congenital lipomatous overgrowth, vascular malformations, epidermal nevi, and spinal/skeletal anomalies and/or scoliosis (CLOVES) syndrome. J Pediatr Adolesc Gynecol 2019;32(6): 648–50.
42. Smits PJ, Konczyk DJ, Sudduth CL, et al. Endothelial MAP2K1 mutations in arteriovenous malformation activate the RAS/MAPK pathway. Biochem Biophys Res Commun 2020;529(2):450–4.
43. Uller W, Alomari AI, Richter GT. Arteriovenous malformations. Semin Pediatr Surg 2014;23(4):203–7.
44. Couto JA, Huang AY, Konczyk DJ, et al. Somatic MAP2K1 mutations are associated with extracranial arteriovenous malformation. Am J Hum Genet 2017;100(3):546–54.
45. Nikolaev SI, Vetiska S, Bonilla X, et al. Somatic activating KRAS mutations in arteriovenous malformations of the brain. N Engl J Med 2018;378(3):250–61.
46. Lekwuttikarn R, Lim YH, Admani S, et al. Genotype-guided medical treatment of an arteriovenous malformation in a child. JAMA Dermatol 2019;155(2): 256–7.
47. Edwards EA, Phelps AS, Cooke D, et al. Monitoring arteriovenous malformation response to genotype-targeted therapy. Pediatrics 2020;146(3).
48. Xie F, Ling L, van Dam H, et al. TGF-β signaling in cancer metastasis. Acta Biochim Biophys Sin (Shanghai) 2018;50(1):121–32.
49. Miyazono K, Katsuno Y, Koinuma D, et al. Intracellular and extracellular TGF-β signaling in cancer: some recent topics. Front Med 2018;12(4):387–411.
50. Keppler-Noreuil KM, Parker VE, Darling TN, et al. Somatic overgrowth disorders of the PI3K/AKT/mTOR pathway & therapeutic strategies. Am J Med Genet C Semin Med Genet 2016;172(4):402–21.
51. Ranieri C, Di Tommaso S, Loconte DC, et al. In vitro efficacy of ARQ 092, an allosteric AKT inhibitor, on primary fibroblast cells derived from patients with PIK3CA-related overgrowth spectrum (PROS). Neurogenetics 2018;19(2):77–91.
52. Suzuki Y, Enokido Y, Yamada K, et al. The effect of rapamycin, NVP-BEZ235, aspirin, and metformin on PI3K/AKT/mTOR signaling pathway of PIK3CA-related overgrowth spectrum (PROS). Oncotarget 2017;8(28):45470–83.

Evolving Landscape of Systemic Therapy for Pediatric Atopic Dermatitis

Mary Kate Lockhart, MD*, Elaine C. Siegfried, MD

KEYWORDS

• Atopic dermatitis • Quality of life • Comorbidities • Biologic • Dupilumab • Safety

KEY POINTS

- Atopic dermatitis (AD) is a common, chronic inflammatory skin disease associated with type 2 T-helper (TH2) dysfunction.
- People with AD are at increased risk for multiple atopic morbidities, including allergic rhinitis, allergic conjunctivitis, asthma, and eosinophilic gastrointestinal disease.
- Dupilumab is the first biologic agent approved by the United States Food and Drug Administration that downregulates TH2 inflammation.
- Dupilumab is currently licensed to treat AD in adults, adolescents, and children down to age 6 years, with ongoing trials including younger children and infants to age 6 months.
- Optimal treatment of AD remains a significant unmet medical need, but multiple new drugs, targeting a range of proinflammatory molecules, hold promise for safer and more effective treatment.

INTRODUCTION

Atopic dermatitis (AD) is a chronic, relapsing inflammatory skin disease that occurs in a characteristic distribution, with associated xerosis and intense pruritus. AD affects approximately 15% of children in the United States with an annual direct and indirect economic burden of ~$5 billion.[1] Moderate-severe AD is not typically life threatening, but can be enormously life altering, with a significant impact on quality of life, restful sleep, school performance, as well as psychological and emotional well-being.

AD is primarily a disease of childhood, with onset at age less than 2 years in the most cases. The condition spontaneously improves in many children with mild-moderate AD, but can be lifelong in those with more severe disease. The pathophysiology of AD is believed to result from a complex interplay of impaired skin barrier function, environmental factors, colonizing and pathogenic microbes, and immune dysregulation, with enhanced type 2 T-helper (TH2) responses and increases in corresponding inflammatory cytokines. Onset in infancy may be developmentally related to more active type 2 immune function in infants, followed by spontaneous improvement in childhood as normal immune maturation biases toward type 1 immune expression.[13] However, for children with moderate-severe AD, the disease is more likely to persist into adulthood. The phenotypic result is erythema, induration, lichenification, and excoriation. There is also an association with subsequent development of other atopic morbidities including asthma, allergic rhinitis, food allergies, and eosinophilic gastrointestinal disease.[2] Immune and skin barrier dysfunction contribute to relative cutaneous anergy, manifest as chronic colonization with *Staphylococcus aureus* and more frequent infections with a variety of microbes, including group A *Streptococcus*, dermatophyte, molluscum, and herpes simplex.

Division of Dermatology, Department of Pediatrics, Cardinal Glennon Children's Hospital, St. Louis University School of Medicine, 1465 South Grand Boulevard, St. Louis, MO 63104, USA
* Corresponding author.
E-mail address: Marykate.k.lockhart@health.slu.edu

Dermatol Clin 40 (2022) 137–143
https://doi.org/10.1016/j.det.2021.12.002
0733-8635/22/© 2021 Elsevier Inc. All rights reserved.

These infections may be occult, lacking the clinical features that characterize similar infections in nonatopic hosts.

In infants and toddlers, AD presents with pruritic, red, weeping or scaly, and crusted lesions more prominent on the extensor surfaces of limbs and on the trunk, face, and scalp, classically sparing the diaper area (**Fig. 1**). Prominent sparing of the nose ("lightbulb sign or Yamamoto sign") has also been described. In older children and adolescents, AD typically affects antecubital and popliteal fossae, with frequent involvement of the volar aspect of the wrists, ankles, and neck (**Fig. 2**). Histologically, AD demonstrates features that include epidermal spongiosis and parakeratosis, and superficial dermal perivascular infiltrate (**Fig. 3**).

Low socioeconomic status, which disproportionately impacts black children, limits access to specialty care, and this has a negative effect on management of children with AD, contributing to poor disease control. A higher percentage of skin changes are also more persistent and dramatic in children with darker skin types, especially lichenification and hyperpigmentation. Secondary tinea may also be more common in African American children who are at higher risk for tinea capitis.[3]

MANAGEMENT

Until there is a cure for AD, management focuses on relieving symptoms and preventing flares while minimizing therapeutic risks. Mounting evidence suggests that early control of inflammation may support normalized immune maturation and decrease long-term risk of extracutaneous atopy. Variables that impact optimal choice of treatment include patient preference and ability, safety and efficacy, cost and access, and comorbidities.

Treatment strategies are aimed at restoring impaired barrier function, reducing itch, minimizing inflammation, recognizing and treating infection, and promoting restful sleep.[4] Approach to therapy can be organized in a stepwise fashion, based on disease severity (see **Fig. 3**).[5] Initial therapy includes bleach baths, avoidance of complex topical allergens. Topical corticosteroids (TCS) have been used first line since their discovery in the 1950s. Widespread and long-term use has informed safety. Because children have a higher ratio of body surface area to weight, safe and effective use of TCS requires monitoring to avoid risks associated with percutaneous absorption, including adrenal suppression. Long-term use of TCS is safest when applied in the morning and no more than an average of once every other day, using a product with the lowest effective potency and in supervised quantities.[6] Maintenance therapy with a TCS-sparing agent is added for children who require daily medication. Choices include topical calcineurin inhibitors (tacrolimus and pimecrolimus) and crisaborole, an inhibitor of type 4 phosphodiesterase (PDE4); however, access to these medications is often limited by payers, often based on labeling for children aged 2 years or greater.

TRADITIONAL SYSTEMIC THERAPY

Until 2017, the only systemic treatments US Food and Drug Administration (FDA)-approved to treat AD were corticosteroids. Only after decades of experience were the risks of this approach recognized to outweigh the benefits. The standard-of-care alternative for patients with severe disease requiring long-term therapy was off-label treatment with immunomodulating and immune suppressive medications. Choices include methotrexate, cyclosporine, mycophenolate mofetil, and azathioprine. Each of these medications has the potential for drug-specific side effects. All require regular laboratory monitoring for associated toxicity.

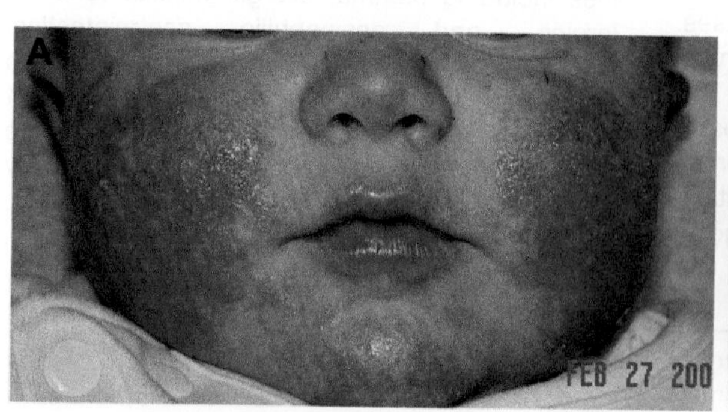

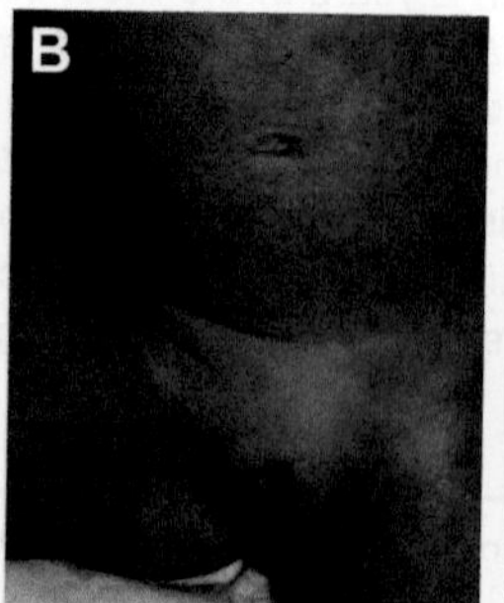

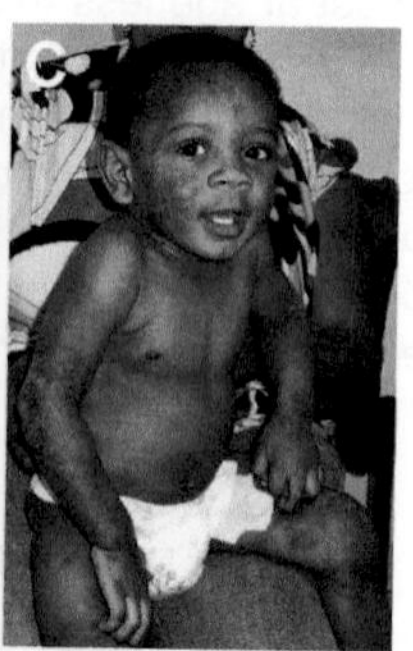

Fig. 1. (*A*) Erythema, edema, and crusting on the face of an infant. Note "Yamamoto sign" sparing of the nose. (*B*) Prominent diaper area sparing is characteristic of atopic dermatitis in infants. (*C*) This infant with atopic dermatitis has involvement of his extensor extremities and face as well as Yamamoto sign.

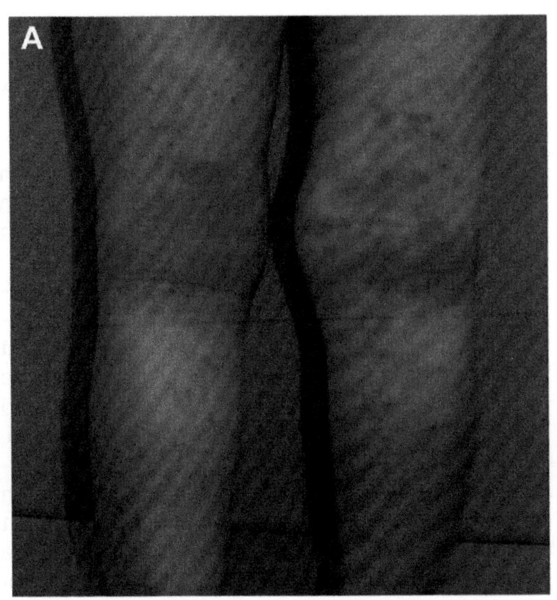

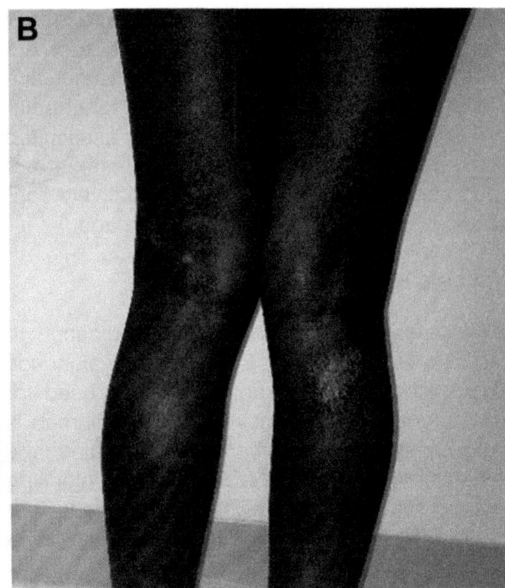

Fig. 2. (*A* and *B*) Scaly and lichenified plaques involving the popliteal fossae are characteristic of AD; associated hyperpigmentation is most prominent in skin of color.

Methotrexate and cyclosporine are the most widely used agents, cyclosporine for its rapid onset and methotrexate for ease of administration and relatively better safety profile. Although the well-established mechanism of action for high-dose methotrexate as cancer chemotherapy is to inhibit dihydrofolate reductase, impairing DNA synthesis, the pharmacologic basis of low-dose methotrexate in controlling inflammation is unclear. Weekly administered, low-dose methotrexate is generally well-tolerated. The most common adverse effects, nausea and abdominal

AD Severity informs customized stepped therapy

	Mild	Moderate	Severe
Maintenance	**Skin care** Daily bath (bleach optional) Liberal, frequent moisturizer use **Trigger avoidance** Irritants, potential topical allergens, low ambient humidity **Consider comorbidities**	**Add bleach baths, wet wraps** **Maintenance topical corticosteroid-sparing medication*** • Twice daily • Monitor quantities **Intermittent TCS** • Medium potency • 15 d per mo • Monitor quantities	**Specialist referral** **Consider comorbidities** **Short-term aggressive treatment** • Wet wraps • Hospitalization **Phototherapy** **Systemic immunosuppressants**** • Methotrexate • Cyclosporine • Mycophenolate mofetil • Azathioprine **Dupilumab**
Flare	**TCS** • Low-to-medium potency • PRN up to 15 d per mo • Monitor quantities	**TCS** • Medium-to-high potency	**Other considerations** • Non-adherence • Infection • Contact allergy • Misdiagnosis

TCS=topical corticosteroid

*topical calcineurin inhibitors (tacrolimus, pimecrolimus), crisaborole, ruxolitinib, vitamin D analogs

***used off-label for AD*

Fig. 3. Stepwise treatment approach for AD. Patients with moderate-severe AD whose skin disease cannot be adequately controlled using adjunctive skin care and optimal amounts of TCS and topical calcineurin inhibitors are candidates for systemic treatment or phototherapy. PRN, as needed; TCS, topical corticosteroids. (*Adapted from* Boguniewicz M, Fonacier L, Guttman-Yassky E, et al. Atopic dermatitis yardstick: practical recommendations for an evolving therapeutic landscape. Ann Allergy Asthma Immunol 2018;120(1):10–22.e2.)

pain, can be mitigated by folic acid, using doses of 1 to 5 mg per day. Standard monitoring for patients on methotrexate is with baseline and follow-up blood tests for hepatic and renal function, and hematologic parameters for associated macrocytosis and leukopenias. Methotrexate is an abortifacient and teratogen, so relatively contraindicated in females of childbearing age.[7]

DUPILUMAB

Development of the first biologic medication to specifically target type 2 immune dysfunction addressed a significant unmet medical need for patients with moderate-severe AD. Dupilumab is a fully human monoclonal antibody that binds the interleukin (IL)-4 receptor alpha subunit, blocking signaling via IL-4 and IL-13, key cytokines that trigger TH2 inflammation. Dupilumab was FDA approved for adults in March 2017, for adolescents in March 2019, and in children down to age 6 years in May 2020. Ongoing clinical trials include children with moderate-severe AD as young as 6 months. Dupilumab is also approved for treatment of asthma in patients down to age 12 years, and for allergic sinusitis with rhinopolyposis in adults.[8]

Dupilumab is administered subcutaneously, with a loading dose, to accelerate onset of response, followed by maintenance dosing every other week or once per month, depending on weight. Data from long-term clinical trials in adults support the safety of dosing as often as once a week, or as infrequently as once a month. It is available in 200- and 300-mg prefilled syringe and 300-mg autoinjector. Labeled dosing for pediatric patients is weight-group based.

Labeled dosing for dupilumab in AD

- 60 kg or more: 600 mg loading dose and 300 mg every other week
- 30 to less than 60 kg: 400 mg loading dose and 200 mg every other week
- Less than 30 kg: 600 mg loading dose and 300 mg every 4 weeks

Other dosing regimens, including a 200 mg load followed by 100 mg every other week for children weighing less than 30 kg and 600 mg load followed by 300 mg once per month for children weighing greater than 30 kg, were studied, but found to be less effective. Individual pharmacokinetics vary, but suggest that younger children may require higher weight-based doses.[14] Higher doses have not been associated with increased adverse effects. Optimal dosing for younger children is under investigation, but weight-based loading doses as high as 15 mg/kg and maintenance doses up to 10 mg/kg every other week have been used. The drug is supplied in 2-syringe units. Refrigerated storage is required to maintain stability. Each box of syringes is marked with a temperature-sensitive label to detect warming.

On-label initial dosing is recommended. With time, some children whose skin has cleared on bimonthly injections may be maintained with less-frequent, monthly injections.

In contrast to the other systemic agents, treatment with dupilumab does not require routine laboratory monitoring. Limited data suggest that dupilumab has no impact on humoral response to immunization. The standard class-labeled recommendation is to avoid live vaccines. Anaphylaxis has been rarely reported, so as a precaution, the first injection is usually performed in the office along with injection training. Subsequent injections are most often done by a caregiver in the home, but some families prefer the assistance of in-office administration. Itch and associated excoriation generally improve within 2 weeks of starting treatment, followed by the signs of eczema: induration, erythema, and scale.

Common adverse effects recognized during clinical trials include injection site reactions and ocular surface disease (most often conjunctivitis, but also keratitis). Eye inflammation may be more common, and more symptomatic in patients with preexisting ocular inflammation, and in adults. Worsening skin inflammation, especially on the face, has been more well-recognized postmarketing. The cause of facial inflammation is not well understood, and been attributed to a variety of triggers, including *Malassezia* colonization, psoriasis, and allergic contact dermatitis. Needle phobia is a common concern for children, but this typically improves with time.

Antidrug antibodies were detected in a small number of study subjects at baseline, and an increasing number over time. However, the clinical significance of these antibodies remains a subject of investigation, including recognition of antibodies considered neutralizing and nonneutralizing.

Ongoing long-term trials in children with AD suggest a mitigating impact of early treatment with dupilumab on the natural history of the disease. Dupilumab is also under investigation for a variety of other atopic conditions, including eosinophilic esophagitis and to enhance the efficacy of oral peanut immunotherapy; this offers hope that a safe and effective drug will one day be available to target the systemic inflammation underlying atopy and fill a significant unmet need for a single medication that can treat, or possibly prevent, the

Table 1
Biologic agents in development

	≥2 y	
Agent	Administration route	Trial Phase for AD
JAK1 inhibitor		
Abrocitinib	Oral	3 (≥12 y)
Aryl hydrocarbon receptor agonist		
Tapinarof	Topical	2 (≥12 y)
PDE4 inhibitors		
Lotamast	Topical	2a (≥2 y)

constellation of atopic comorbidities that begin in childhood.[2]

Insight into the duration of therapy will require additional information from ongoing long-term trials. However, in the author's experience a small proportion of patients have been able to discontinue dupilumab without relapse for as long as 2 years. Meanwhile, our approach is to begin by tapering treatment (dose amount or dosing interval up to 1 month) only after complete clearing for a minimum of 3 months. Discontinuation should be considered if clearing is maintained after a minimum 3-month taper.

Although the impressive efficacy and safety has been proved in large clinical trials, insurance coverage for dupilumab remains a significant barrier to access. Health care providers prescribing dupilumab are frequently challenged by need for prior authorization and subsequent denial. Before formal FDA approval for children, a retrospective analysis of patterns of insurance denials for pediatric patients found that lack of pediatric-specific labeling was the most common reason for denial. In some cases, step-edit requirements ironically demanded off-label use of immunosuppressant drugs.[9] Completion of phase 3 trials and labeling for use in children has had a positive impact on access.

HORIZON

The pipeline is robust for new drugs to treat AD, as well as other atopic conditions. Although AD is primarily a disease of children, pediatric clinical trials always follow trials in adults, and always include fewer subjects. Long-term, open-label extension studies and data from use for other pediatric indications will help inform the relative risks and benefits for each product and pathway.

Several monoclonal antibodies are in development that largely target the TH2 pathway. Tralokinumab and lebrikizumab bind circulating IL-13, and ASLAN004 binds the IL-13 subunit receptor

Table 2
Biologic agents in development

	≥18 y	
Agent	Administration route	Trial phase for AD
Monoclonal antibodies (target)		
Tezepelumab (TSLP)	SQ	2a completed
Afuco (IL-31)	SQ	Ib completed
Nemolizumab (IL-31)	SQ	2 completed
GBR 830 (O × 40)	IV	2
Fezakinumab (IL-22)	IV	2 Published
Lebrikizumab (IL-13)	SQ	3
Tralokinumab (IL-13)	SQ	3
MOR106 (IL-17C)	IV	2 failed
Pitrakinra (IL-4)	SQ	2a completed
Ligelizumab (IgE)	SQ	2 completed
JAK inhibitors		
Gusacitinib (JAK-SYK)	Oral	2b
Baricitinib (JAK 1/2)	Oral	2b completed
Upadacitinib (JAK 1)	Oral	2
Ruxolitinib (JAK 1/2)	Topical	2 completed
PDE 4 inhibitors		
Roflumilast (ARQ-151)	Topical	2a

with downstream effects that are similar, but not identical to, dupilumab IL-4 receptor subunit blockade.[9] Nemolizumab binds IL-31 receptor A, known to play an important role in the pathogenesis of itch.[10] A phase 2 trial in adults with AD yielded improved itch, but less clinical improvement in the signs of eczema, arguing against the historic description of AD as "the itch that rashes."

Another less specific target for the treatment of AD is Janus kinases (JAK). This family of cytoplasmic protein tyrosine kinases is critical for nuclear signal transduction. JAK inhibitors (sometimes referred to as "jakinibs") are small molecules that offer the advantage of oral as well as topical administration, and likely more rapid response than the current biologics under investigation. A disadvantage is a likely greater impact on immune function, with a theoretically higher risk of infection or carcinogenicity with long-term use. Increased risk of venous thromboembolism is another concern.[11] Together, these risks prompted a new class black box warning for all JAK inhibitors, topical and systemic. The different products vary with regard to selectivity for the 4 recognized JAK targets, JAKs 1, 2, and 3, and TYK2.[12] Three JAK inhibitors have been FDA approved to treat a variety of inflammatory disorders, beginning with tofacitinib (Xeljanz), for adults with rheumatoid arthritis (RA), psoriatic arthritis, and ulcerative colitis, as well as children with juvenile idiopathic arthritis weighing as little as 10 kg. Upadacitinib (Rinvoq) and baricitinib (Olumiant) are labeled to treat RA in adults, but are under investigation for treating AD. Abrocitinib is a selective JAK1 inhibitor in clinical trials for moderate-to-severe AD in adults and adolescents. Clinical trials in adults and adolescents with mild-to-moderate AD are ongoing for ruxolitinib, a topical JAK1/2 inhibitor.

Other agents in development include biologics targeting TSLP (thymic stromal lymphopoietin), IL-4, IL-22, IL-17 C, IgE, PDE4, and aryl hydrocarbon receptor (see tables). Most clinical trials for moderate-severe AD have not included children younger than 12 years to date. However, the pipeline is robust, so the treatment paradigm for AD is sure to evolve (**Tables 1** and **2**).

CLINICS CARE POINTS

- AD is a chronic disease with significant impact on quality of life.
- Treatment of mild and moderate AD begins with skin care and topical medication.
- A proactive approach is more effective than reactive treatment.
- Proactive treatment is stepwise and based on disease severity and associated morbidities.
- Off-label use of oral immunosuppressant and immunomodulating medications (most often methotrexate or cyclosporine) have been the only options until recently. The following factors support the need for dupilumab therapy in pediatric patients:
  - Moderate-severe AD
  - Extracutaneous atopic morbidities (asthma, rhinitis, eosinophilic gastrointestinal disease, food allergy)
  - High total IgE
  - Strong family history of atopy

DISCLOSURES

Dr M.K. Lockhart has nothing to disclose.

Dr E.C. Siegfried:

AI Therapeutics: contracted research.

ASLAN Pharmaceuticals: consultant fees

Boehringer Ingelheim: consulting fees

Incyte: consulting fees

Regeneron: consulting fees, honoraria; fees to SSM/SLU related to sponsoring clinical trials.

Sanofi Genzyme: consulting fees, honoraria.

UCB: DSMB, consulting fees

Abbvie: consulting fees

Verrica: consulting fees, honoraria; fees to SSM/SLU related to sponsoring a clinical trial.

Leo: consulting fees, DSMB.

Novan: consulting fees; DSMB.

Novartis: consulting fees

Pfizer: consulting fee; DSMB; grant funding to support 2020–2022 Peds Derm Fellow.

Pierre Fabre: consulting fee; fees to SSM/SLU related to sponsoring a clinical trial.

Janssen: PI, fees to SSM/SLU related to sponsoring a clinical trial.

Lilly: fees to SSM/SLU related to sponsoring a clinical trial.

REFERENCES

1. Sidbury R, Siegfried, EC. Atopic dermatitis. Chapter 8.1.
2. Siegfried EC, Igelman S, Jaworski JC, et al. Use of dupilumab in pediatric atopic dermatitis: access, dosing, and implications for managing severe atopic dermatitis. Pediatr Dermatol 2019;36:172–6. https://doi.org/10.1111/pde.13707.
3. Siegfried EC, Paller AS, Mina-Osorio P, et al. Effects of variations in access to care for children with

atopic dermatitis. BMC Dermatol 2020;20:24. https://doi.org/10.1186/s12895-020-00114-x.
4. Ramirez FD, Chen S, Langan SM, et al. Association of atopic dermatitis with sleep quality in children. JAMA Pediatr 2019;173:e190025.
5. Boguniewicz M, Fonacier L, Guttman-Yassky E, et al. Atopic dermatitis yardstick: Practical recommendations for an evolving therapeutic landscape. Ann Allergy Asthma Immunol 2018;120:10–22.e2.
6. Eichenfield LF, Tom WL, Berger TG, et al. Guidelines of care for the management of atopic dermatitis: section 2. Management and treatment of atopic dermatitis with topical therapies. J Am Acad Dermatol 2014;71(1):116–32.
7. Igelman S, Kurta AO, Sheikh U, et al. Off-label use of dupilumab for pediatric patients with atopic dermatitis: a multicenter retrospective review. J Am Acad Dermatol 2020;82(2):407–11. https://doi.org/10.1016/j.jaad.2019.10.010.
8. Wang CY, Zheng RRC, Doerrer ZA, et al. Health care regulation, the Food and Drug Administration (FDA), and access to medicine: our experience with dupilumab for children. J Am Acad Dermatol 2020;82(6):1568–9. https://doi.org/10.1016/j.jaad.2020.01.019.
9. Siegels D, Heratizadeh A, Abraham S, et al, European Academy of Allergy, Clinical Immunology Atopic Dermatitis Guideline Group. Systemic treatments in the management of atopic dermatitis: a systematic review and meta-analysis. Allergy 2021;76(4):1053–76. https://doi.org/10.1111/all.14631.
10. Ruzicka T, Hanifin JM, Furue M, et al. Anti-interleukin-31 receptor a antibody for atopic dermatitis. N Engl J Med 2017;376:826–35. https://doi.org/10.1056/NEJMoa1606490.
11. Cohen SB. JAK inhibitors and VTE risk: how concerned should we be? Nat Rev Rheumatol 2021;17:133–4. https://doi.org/10.1038/s41584-021-00575-5.
12. McInnes IB, Byers NL, Higgs RE, et al. Comparison of baricitinib, upadacitinib, and tofacitinib mediated regulation of cytokine signaling in human leukocyte subpopulations. Arthritis Res Ther 2019;21:183. https://doi.org/10.1186/s13075-019-1964-1.
13. Simon AK, Hollander GA, McMichael A. Evolution of the immune system in humans from infancy to old age. Proc Biol Sci 2015;282(1821):20143085. https://doi.org/10.1098/rspb.2014.3085.
14. Paller AS, Siegfried EC, Simpson EL, et al. A phase 2, open-label study of single-dose dupilumab in children aged 6 months to <6 years with severe uncontrolled atopic dermatitis: pharmacokinetics, safety and efficacy. J Eur Acad Dermatol Venereol 2021;35(2):464–75. https://doi.org/10.1111/jdv.16928.

Clinical Decisions in Pediatric Psoriasis

A Practical Approach to Systemic Therapy

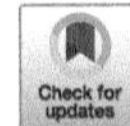

Jennifer Ornelas, MD, Kelly M. Cordoro, MD*

KEYWORDS

• Psoriasis • Pediatric psoriasis • Psoriasis treatments • Systemic treatments • Biologics • DMARDS

KEY POINTS

- When deciding whether to start a systemic treatment for pediatric psoriasis patients, providers should take into account objective and subjective severity, comorbidities, potential triggers, and the functional and psychological impact of the psoriasis.
- All available systemic and biologic treatments for psoriasis can and should be considered for moderate to severe pediatric psoriasis patients.
- Systemic treatments include two main categories: conventional treatments, including acitretin, methotrexate, and cyclosporine, and biologic treatments including TNFα inhibitors, IL-12/23 inhibitors, IL-17 inhibitors, and the PDE-4 inhibitor, apremilast.
- Providers should create a tailored approach for each patient when selecting a systemic therapy, taking into account disease factors and drug characteristics such as lab monitoring, formulation, method and frequency of administration, feasibility, cost and patient preferences.

INTRODUCTION

The management of moderate to severe pediatric psoriasis is multi-faceted and guided by a holistic consideration of several interrelated factors. Type of psoriasis, triggers, physical and psychological impact, comorbid conditions, patient age, family preferences, clinician experience and treatment efficacy, safety and cost all factor in. The chronicity of psoriasis and its tendency toward unpredictable periods of remission and relapse complicates decisions about initiation and continuation of systemic therapy. There are some clinical situations that indicate a specific treatment, but in most cases, there is therapeutic flexibility and approach is individualized.

Kids with psoriasis in visible locations may be teased or bullied and choose to self-isolate. The impact on self-esteem and identity formation can be significant, and adequately treating children of all ages to prevent downstream negative consequences of psoriasis is critical. Historically, children have been under-treated[1]; this may be due in part to access to medicines and fear of side effects on a growing child. Now more than ever, more medicines are being tested for safety and efficacy in children, and physicians no longer have to rely on adult studies to inform treatment choices for children. Given the potentially high stakes of chronic inflammation, including the observed risk of cardiovascular disease (CVD) in young psoriatic adults, the risks of under-treated severe psoriasis are likely far greater than the risks of its treatments. Choice between phototherapy, conventional systemic and targeted biologic therapy is ideally tailored to the clinical scenario and agreed upon by the clinician, patient and caregivers.

This article is intended to provide a practical clinical framework for management of the subset of children with widespread, severe or recalcitrant psoriasis who require treatment with systemic

Department of Dermatology, University of California, San Francisco School of Medicine, 1701 Divisadero Street, San Francisco, CA 94143, USA
* Corresponding author.
E-mail address: kelly.cordoro@ucsf.edu

Dermatol Clin 40 (2022) 145–166
https://doi.org/10.1016/j.det.2021.12.003
0733-8635/22/© 2022 Elsevier Inc. All rights reserved.

medications. Though pediatric-specific data on pathophysiology, risk factors, triggers, comorbidities, natural history and therapeutics are limited, there is a small body of evidence that can be combined with robust clinical experience to guide medical decision making. We offer real life case examples to illustrate the use of various therapies and the principles discussed herein.

Psoriasis results from an auto-amplifying inflammatory cascade involving the innate and adaptive immune system. Historically, systemic therapies used to treat psoriasis have relied upon broad and relatively non-specific immune suppression (methotrexate, cyclosporine) and reduction of keratinocyte proliferation (retinoids). The evolving understanding of the pathogenic role of activated T cells driving inflammatory pathways that involve cytokines such as TNFα, IL-17, IL-12 and IL-23 has led to development of selective inhibitors of these pathways. Preliminary data have shown that pediatric psoriasis may be uniquely mediated by IL-22[2] though currently there are no commercially available IL-22 inhibitors. The regulatory pathways targeted by treatments produce both therapeutic efficacy and the potential for mechanism-based adverse effects. For example, a broad-acting conventional therapy such as methotrexate is effective at reducing psoriasis but may also cause bone marrow suppression. Similarly, IL-17 inhibitors effectively treat psoriasis but increase the risk of mucocutaneous candidiasis given IL-17's role in defense against this extracellular organism.[3,4] A clear understanding of each medication's mechanism of action and the potential for mechanism-based side effects is an important aspect of drug selection.

Illustrative Case: Case 1

An otherwise healthy 10-years-old boy is referred to clinic for severe psoriasis. He has had localized plaques for 5 years that recently became widespread and failed to respond to topical and phototherapy. He has missed 4 weeks of school due to the severity of his psoriasis. Father has psoriasis and mother has vitiligo. Parents are divorced. During the encounter, his father is frustrated and his mother is tearful. Examination reveals a shy boy unwilling to make eye contact. He is lying uncomfortably on the table with legs in a flexed position. He has widespread plaques and near-erythroderma involving the scalp, face, trunk, extremities, genitals, palms and soles (**Fig. 1**). There are erosions of the flexures and painful fissures on the palms and soles. How should we manage this patient?

THE SYSTEMIC THERAPY TOOL BOX

All systemic therapies may be considered for children presenting with severe psoriasis. A simple framework for thinking about the options divides them into two broad categories: "tried and true" and "new and novel." (**Fig. 2**) Tried and true treatments are the oldies but goodies; those medications including methotrexate, cyclosporine and acitretin that are devoid of rigorous placebo-controlled randomized clinical trial-based evidence but have been used successfully and safely for decades for pediatric psoriasis. None are FDA approved for this indication. Phototherapy, primarily NB-UVB, is another "tried and true" treatment for a subset of children with moderate to severe psoriasis for whom it is accessible and feasible.

The "new and novel" treatments have been developed more recently and selectively target components of the inflammatory cascade. These include monoclonal antibodies against TNFα, IL-12/23, IL-23 and IL-17, and the small molecule phosphodiesterase 4 (PDE4) inhibitor, apremilast. Fortunately, robust clinical trial data are accumulating, and several targeted therapies are U.S. FDA-approved for children with psoriasis including the anti-TNFα agent etanercept (4 years and older), the anti-IL-12/23 agent ustekinumab (6 years and older) and the anti-IL-17 agents ixekizumab (6 years and older) and secukinumab (6 years and older). Several additional targeted therapies are under evaluation in pediatric trials. (**Tables 1** and **2**).

ASSESSMENT OF SEVERITY

When selecting a treatment regimen for a child with psoriasis, consider the overall disease burden using both objective and subjective measures. Objective measures such as body surface area (BSA) assess the extent of involvement such that the higher the BSA, the more severe the psoriasis. Mild is defined as less than 3% BSA, moderate is 3% to 10% BSA and greater than 10% BSA is considered severe. Another objective severity instrument used primarily in research as opposed to clinical practice is the Psoriasis Area and Severity Index (PASI). This tool measures the severity and extent of psoriasis by accounting for intensity of redness, scaling, and plaque thickness and area of involvement.

Subjective measures can be powerful tools to gain insight into the disease burden beyond the skin including impact on quality of life (QOL). The goal of subjective inquiry is to identify functional impairment and less tangible effects such as

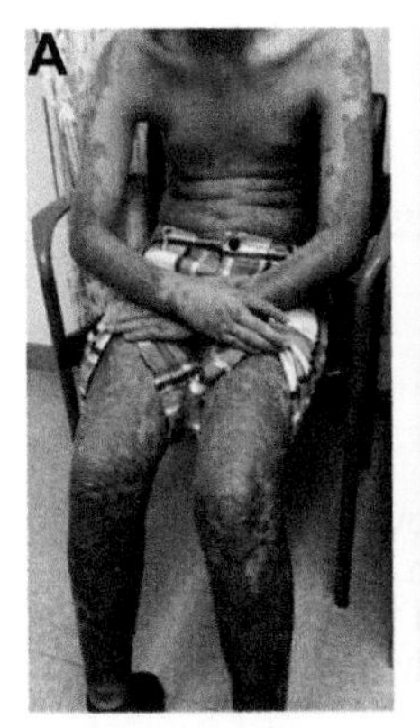

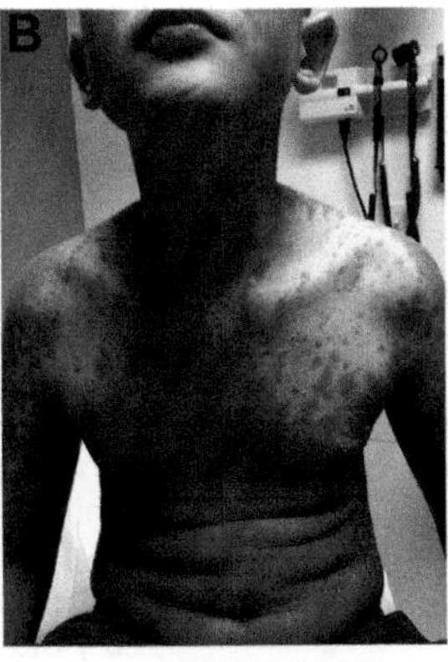

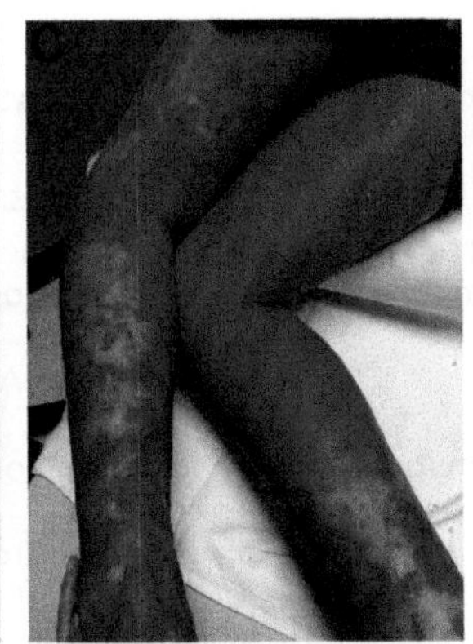

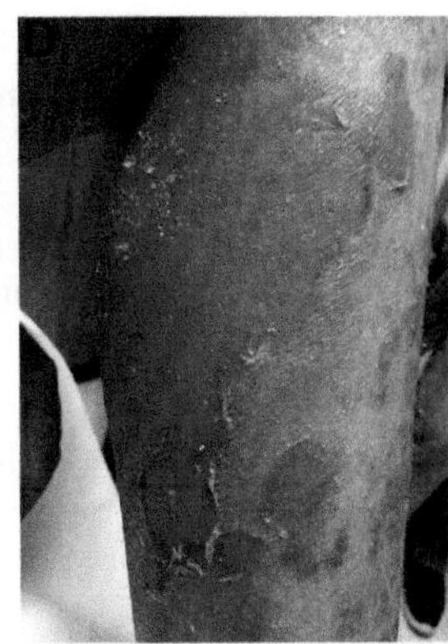

Fig. 1. Illustrative Case 1. 10-year-old boy with severe psoriasis. (*A–D*) On exam he is found to have widespread plaques and near erythroderma with involvement of the scalp, face, trunk, extremities, genitals, palms and soles. There are erosions of the flexures and painful fissures on the palms and soles.

embarrassment, shame, bullying and withdrawal. Assessments of subjective severity can be made through simple open-ended questions or via formal questionnaires. The Children's Dermatology Life Quality Index (CDLQI) is a 10-question survey that has been validated for pediatric psoriasis and assesses QOL for patients ages 4 through 16 years by addressing variables such as itch, sleep, hygiene, impact on relationships and activities, and treatment efficacy.[5] The potential for negative downstream impacts of subjectively severe psoriasis on health, education, recreation, occupation and relationships is substantial. Consider an adolescent patient with psoriasis involving 2% BSA. Objectively, this is mild, but if the limited BSA involves the face, hands or genitals, this may prompt shame and bullying due to the visible location, inability to participate in sports, and embarrassment leading to social isolation. Pediatric patients, especially in early adolescence, confront significant challenges to self-esteem and identity formation based on comparison with peers and the idealized social construct of beauty even in the absence of skin pathology. The presence of skin disease may negatively influence psychosocial development and adjustment and increase the rates of maladjustment and mental health disorders.[6–8] Accounting for the additional impact of psoriasis on psychosocial development and wellbeing is critical as management plans are developed. The modified Cutaneous Body Image questionnaire can be used to capture an adolescent's satisfaction with their skin, hair and nails and develop shared management goals.[9]

Tools to manage severe psoriasis in pediatric patients

Tried and True
Methotrexate
Cyclosporine
Acitretin
Phototherapy

New and Novel
TNF inhibitors
IL-12/23 inhibitors
IL-17 inhibitors

Fig. 2. "Tried and True" and "New and Novel" treatments for severe psoriasis in pediatric patients.

Table 1
List of FDA and EMA approvals of biologics for pediatric psoriasis

Class	Drug	FDA Approval	EMA Approval
Anti- TNFα	Etanercept	≥4 y old	≥ 6 y old
	Adalimumab	Not approved for psoriasis in children Approved for JIA in ages ≥ 2 y old	≥4 y old
	Infliximab	Not approved for psoriasis in children Approved for Crohn's and Ulcerative Colitis in ages ≥ 6 y old	Not approved for psoriasis in children Approved for Crohn's and Ulcerative Colitis in ages ≥ 6 y old
	Certolizumab	Not approved for psoriasis in children[a]	Not approved for psoriasis in children
IL-17 inhibitors	Ixekizumab	≥6 y old	≥6 y old and ≥ 25 kg
	Secukinumab	≥6 y old	≥6 y old
	Brodalumab	Not approved for psoriasis in children[a]	Not approved for psoriasis in children
IL-12/23 inhibitor	Ustekinumab	≥ 6 y old	≥6 y old
IL-23 inhibitor	Guselkumab	Not approved for psoriasis in children[a]	Not approved for psoriasis in children
	Risankizumab	Not approved for psoriasis in children[a]	Not approved for psoriasis in children
PDE4 inhibitor	Apremilast	Not approved for psoriasis in children[a]	Not approved for psoriasis in children

Abbreviations: EMA, european medicines agency; FDA, united states food and drug administration.
[a] There are ongoing phase 3 clinical trial for the approval of these medications in children 6 y and older in the US

THRESHOLD FOR INITIATING SYSTEMIC THERAPY

The threshold for initiating systemic therapy for psoriasis in pediatric patients varies by age and clinical context.

Considerations Based on Age

Neonates, infants and young children

In general, the younger the patient, the more conservative the initial approach. Key considerations for neonates, infants and young children presenting with moderate to severe psoriasis are monogenic conditions and infectious triggers. Viral infections may trigger the immune system in children of all ages, and pharyngeal and anogenital group A β-hemolytic streptococcal infections are associated with the development of guttate and plaque psoriasis.[10–12] Because a subset of children with a streptococcal infection may clear their psoriasis and go into remission,[13] a more conservative initial approach with topical therapy and culture-directed antibiotics is reasonable, with escalation to systemic therapy as indicated. Monogenic autoinflammatory diseases that present with psoriasiform eruptions should also be

Table 2
Summary of systemic therapies in clinical trials for moderate-severe psoriasis in pediatric patients

Class	Medication	ClinicalTrials.gov Identifier	Enrollment
TNFα inhibitor	Certolizumab	NCT04123795	Ages 6–17
IL-23 inhibitor	Guselkumab	NCT03451851	Ages 6–17
	Risankizumab	NCT04435600	Ages 6–17
IL-17 inhibitor	Brodalumab	NCT03240809	Ages 6–17
PDE-4 inhibitor	Apremilast	NCT03701763, NCT04175613	Ages 6–17

considered in this age group. This group of disorders includes deficiency of interleukin-1 receptor antagonist (DIRA), deficiency of interleukin-36 receptor antagonist (DITRA) and caspase recruitment domain family member 14 (CARD14) mediated psoriasis. See below for specific details regarding therapy for these disorders.

School aged children and adolescents

For school aged children and adolescents, in addition to assessing for infection, accounting for both the physical and psychosocial impact of psoriasis is important. Psoriasis has been shown to have a negative impact on the overall quality of life in pediatric patients comparable to that of children with asthma and arthritis, and greater than that of children with diabetes or epilepsy.[14,15] Children with objectively mild disease can have significantly decreased quality of life as related to pain, pruritus and fatigue.[16] Moreover, the physical appearance of psoriasis itself can be viewed as the "worst part" of the disease.[17] Psoriasis can impact the ability of children to function optimally in social situations including school, sports and activities.[15,16,18] Children with psoriasis may be stigmatized and bullied. Adult patients who have an earlier age of onset of psoriasis are more likely to report chronic effects on quality of life and attribute depression to psoriasis compared to adults with similar psoriasis severity but with a later age of onset.[19] It is therefore crucial to assess the psychosocial impact of psoriasis in school aged and especially adolescent patients and take this into account when deciding whether to initiate systemic therapy.

Considerations Based on Comorbidities

The most robust data suggests that mood disorders, obesity, and psoriatic arthritis are the primary comorbidities in children with psoriasis. The presence of one or more of these conditions may influence treatment decisions. A comorbidity screening guidance document for children with psoriasis has been published.[20] In summary, these guidelines suggest that all children with psoriasis should be screened according to the American Academy of Pediatrics (AAP) age-based screening recommendations for all children. Depending on the individual clinical context, additional evaluation may be warranted.

Children with psoriasis have higher rates of mood disorders, especially depression and anxiety, than psoriasis-free peers. This holds true even for younger children ages 8 to 12 years.[15,21] Children with psoriasis and depression are at an increased risk of alcohol and drug use, and even suicidality as they reach late adolescence.[22–24] While neuropsychiatric disorders including depression and suicidality may be related to the social stigmatization of the disease, the cytokine theory suggests that these disturbances may also be intrinsically related.[25] In this context, management of psoriasis requires identification of mood symptoms, low threshold for referral to mental health providers, and adequate treatment of the psoriasis.

Obesity is strongly associated with psoriasis in pediatric patients overall and may be a significant contributor to development of other comorbidities.[26–29] Children with psoriasis and a higher BMI have been shown in some studies to have more severe disease.[28,30] Psoriasis may result in decreased physical activity due to embarrassment related to physical appearance, presence of joint symptoms, or increased pruritus from heat and sweat while exercising.[31] This creates a vicious self-amplifying cycle between obesity and psoriasis. Children with psoriasis are at an increased risk of developing metabolic syndrome-a constellation of conditions that may include obesity, hypertension, hypertriglyceridemia, hypercholesterolemia and insulin resistant diabetes-that increases the risk of cardiovascular disease. The relative contributions to the risk of metabolic syndrome from psoriasis itself versus obesity are unclear, but recent data suggest that obesity is the primary driver.[29,32–34]

The association between the chronic inflammation of psoriasis and the development of cardiovascular disease (CVD) is described as the "psoriatic march." This hypothesis suggests that psoriasis leads to systemic inflammation, insulin resistance, endothelial dysfunction, and atherosclerosis which can ultimately lead to cardiovascular and cerebrovascular disease including myocardial infarction and stroke.[35] Obesity initiates the same inflammatory pathway and risk of CVD. In adult psoriasis patients, disease modifying treatment with methotrexate and TNFα inhibitors for psoriasis has been shown to be cardioprotective and cerebrovascular protective.[36–38] Though it is yet to be determined if early and aggressive treatment of psoriasis in childhood can modify the long-term risk of early onset CVD observed in adult patients, the potential risks of unchecked chronic inflammation should be considered in treatment plans. Patients should be screened for obesity and, when appropriate, metabolic syndrome and other related comorbid conditions. Obese patients should be offered referrals to obesity specialists and lifestyle modification programs. As obesity may increase the risk of adverse effects from methotrexate, cyclosporine and acitretin, these treatments may be less optimal choices for overweight patients.

The presence of juvenile psoriatic arthritis will impact decisions about initiation of systemic therapy. Children with psoriatic arthritis can present with pain and swelling in one or more joints, dactylitis, joint stiffness after rest, limp, enthesitis, or uveitis.[39] There is a bimodal distribution of age of onset with the first peak occurring at 2 to 3 years of age and the second occurring between 10 to 12 years.[20] As opposed to adults, pediatric psoriatic arthritis may often present prior to onset of skin disease.[20,40,41] All children with psoriasis should be screened carefully with a directed review of systems, examination of joints and imaging as indicated. If arthritis is detected or suspected, collaborative management with a pediatric rheumatologist is ideal if available.

WHICH DRUG FOR WHICH PEDIATRIC PATIENT?

All conventional systemic and biologic treatments may be considered for children with moderate to severe psoriasis. In most cases, there is no one "right answer" and treatment decisions must be individualized. However, there are certain clinical scenarios (psoriatic arthritis, monogenic variants, and contraindications) for which specific treatments are warranted.

Children with psoriatic arthritis are at risk for joint damage and impaired function and often require a disease modifying drug such as methotrexate and/or a biologic agent. Patients who are found to have monogenic variants of psoriasis are approached based on the specific disorder. Deficiency of interleukin-1 receptor antagonist (DIRA) is caused by a recessively inherited loss-of-function mutation in the *interleukin-1 receptor antagonist* (*IL-1RN*) gene which results in activation of interleukin-1 (IL-1).[42–46] It is associated with neonatal-onset pustular psoriasis, multifocal osteomyelitis and periostitis, and elevated inflammatory markers.[42–46] Recombinant IL-1 receptor antagonist therapy such as anakinra or canakinumab is lifesaving for these patients.[43] Other monogenic variants presenting with psoriasiform dermatitis do not yet have evidence-based specific therapies though best choices are emerging anecdotally. Deficiency of interleukin-36 receptor antagonist (DITRA) is caused by recessively inherited mutations in *interleukin-36 receptor antagonist* (*IL-36RN*), which result in an unchecked inflammatory cascade.[47,48] It is associated with recurrent episodes of generalized pustular psoriasis (GPP), characteristically in the absence of plaque psoriasis, high fevers, leukocytosis, systemic inflammation and elevated inflammatory markers.[47,48] A uniformly effective treatment for DITRA remains elusive. Published cases have demonstrated clinical response to infliximab,[49] anakinra,[50] ustekinumab,[51,52] and secukinumab[53–56] Recently, an intravenous IL-36 receptor antagonist successfully controlled GPP in adults in the context of *IL36RN* and *CARD14* mutations as well as in GPP patients without known mutations.[57] Caspase recruitment domain family member 14 (*CARD14*)-mediated psoriasiform eruptions result from gain-of-function mutations in *CARD14* with subsequent activation of nuclear factor kappa B (NF-κB) and unchecked inflammation.[58] The spectrum of psoriasis phenotypes related to this genotype includes pustular, plaque, and erythrodermic. These patients often have early-onset psoriasis and psoriasiform eruptions with overlapping features of pityriasis rubra pilaris (PRP).[58–66] Antagonism of IL-12/23 has emerged as a treatment of choice for CARD-14 related psoriasiform eruptions.[67]

Just as certain situations call for specific treatments, there are certain clinical situations in which specific treatments should be avoided. In general, avoid the use of methotrexate in patients with preexisting liver disease including obese patients at risk for fatty liver disease. Methotrexate is renally excreted; thus, MTX should not be prescribed to those with kidney disease or renal failure. Patients with kidney disease or hypertension should also not take cyclosporine given its known renal toxicity and risk of hypertension. Acitretin, a teratogen, should ideally be avoided in females of childbearing potential. While there is no specific age cut-off for females, it is rational to avoid acitretin in females aged 10 years and older since it is stored in the body for up to 3 years when reverse-esterified to etretinate in the presence of alcohol. Oral retinoids should be used with caution in those at risk for familial or acquired dyslipidemia. Lastly, IL-17 inhibitors are ideally avoided in patients with inflammatory bowel disease (IBD) as they may exacerbate IBD.[68]

ADDITIONAL CONSIDERATIONS WHEN SELECTING SYSTEMIC THERAPIES

Beyond the scenarios discussed above, practical considerations and logistics often drive treatment choice including mechanism of action (broad immune suppression vs modulation), monitoring requirements (number and frequency of lab draws), formulation (oral [pills or liquid] vs injectable), feasibility (access to labs, infusion centers, compounding pharmacies), patient acceptability (mode and frequency of administration), availability (coverage, compounded liquids for children unable to swallow capsules) and financial and social costs (price of medicine, lab monitoring, supplies, travel, missed work/wages, missed school/activities). See **Tables 3** and **4** for further details.

"TRIED AND TRUE"
Conventional Systemic Therapies

The "conventional" systemic treatments for psoriasis are those that pre-date monoclonal antibodies against specific cytokines. These drugs include methotrexate, cyclosporine, and acitretin. Phototherapy belongs here as this mode of therapy is often the entry point into systemic therapy. While these "oldies but goodies" may sometimes be overlooked in favor of newer targeted treatments, there are many benefits to their use in selected cases. These medicines have been available for the treatment of psoriasis in pediatric patients for decades and have amassed an abundance of data and experience to support their use. Oral systemics can be combined with other treatments for added benefit. Importantly, these medications are "easy on/easy off" meaning they can be started and stopped relatively easily without necessarily compromising efficacy, safety, or committing the patient to long-term use. This is especially useful, for example, in cases of new or flaring psoriasis in a patient with an identified trigger such as a streptococcal infection whereby the psoriasis may be modified by treating the infection and not require long-term use of an immunosuppressive therapy.

3 Phases of Therapy: Control, Transition, Maintenance.

A practical way to approach the use of conventional systemic therapies is to consider 3 distinct treatment phases: control, transition and maintenance (**Fig. 3**). First, aim to achieve control or clear the psoriasis with the selected agent. Once control is achieved and maintained for a period, transition by tapering immunomodulating medications to the lowest effective dose or stop them. Then, maintain the psoriasis with the lowest effective dose or reduced frequency of administration of the original agent, or with an alternate therapy with a better safety profile such as topicals or phototherapy. The cycle may be repeated upon worsening disease or acute flares whereby the control drug is either restarted, or the maintenance dose escalated to effect, followed by tapering to the lowest effective maintenance dose once control is achieved. The advantage here is the flexibility these medications offer in terms of dosage, combination therapy, and escalation or de-escalation as the situation calls. The drugs may be started and stopped with little risk of loss of efficacy or adverse reaction upon re-initiation and the patient is not committed to long-term use. Combining these agents should be done with attention to potential additive toxicity such as marrow suppression, end-organ effects, and photosensitivity depending on which combinations are used. See **Table 3** for details regarding medication dosage, clinical uses, toxicities and monitoring.

PHOTOTHERAPY

For those with access to phototherapy, narrow band UVB (NB-UVB) phototherapy is a safe and efficacious treatment option for pediatric psoriasis and a subset of patients will achieve remission for up to 2 years.[69] In select cases, NB-UVB can be used with low dose systemic retinoids for a synergistic effect. The addition of NB-UVB therapy (as per Skin Phototype 1 parameters) may provide better control of plaque and pustular psoriasis than acitretin monotherapy.[70] Unfortunately, the use of phototherapy is often limited by logistical hurdles and access. Availability of in-office phototherapy differs across geographic locations and is limited in rural areas.[71] Not all insurers sufficiently cover the cost of in-office treatments and many do not cover home units. Patients and their families must make a significant commitment given the time, cost of travel, and lost wages associated with the recommended three times weekly treatments.

ACITRETIN
Illustrative Case in an Infant: Case 2

An 8 months old infant presents with psoriasis since 3 months of age. Skin biopsy confirms psoriasis and whole exome sequencing (WES) is negative for mutations in the genes causing monogenic forms of psoriasis: *IL-36RN* (DITRA), *IL-1RN* (DIRA), and *CARD14* (CARD-14 Associated Psoriasiform Eruption). He is found to have psoriasis involving approximately 75% BSA with mixed morphology including annular plaques, diffuse scaly pink papules, and scattered pustules. He has a Cushingoid appearance due to over-use of potent topical steroids to wide surface areas over the last several weeks. He is started on acitretin 0.3 mg/kg/d and has a moderate response. The skin improves with dose escalation to 0.5 mg/kg/d and he is nearly clear after 5 weeks (**Fig. 4**).

Acitretin is a non-immunosuppressive treatment for psoriasis and is a good choice for males of all ages, including infants as demonstrated in the case above. Acitretin must be compounded into a liquid formulation for infants and children unable to swallow pills.

It is contraindicated in women of childbearing potential. It is particularly useful for the treatment

Table 3
Dosage, monitoring, and side effects of conventional systemic therapies for psoriasis

Medication	Baseline Labs	Lab Monitoring	Dose and Frequency	Uses	Side Effects	Formulation	Comments
Acitretin	CBC, LFT, fasting lipids, pregnancy test (if appropriate)	LFT and lipids after 1 mo of treatment, then once every 1–3 mo Interval pregnancy tests (if appropriate)	0.1–1 mg/kg/d	Best response with guttate, pustular and palmoplantar psoriasis Can combine with NB-UVB for synergy	Mucocutaneous-xerosis, cheilitis, granulation tissue; transaminitis, hypertriglyceridemia, potential bone effects with chronic use (rare)	Pill May be compounded as liquid	Known teratogen- do not recommend for use in females of childbearing potential Esterified to etretinate and stored in fat for 3 y in the presence of alcohol
Cyclosporine	Blood pressure, CBC, renal function, LFT, fasting lipids, serum magnesium, potassium, and uric acid; HIV for at risk patients. Pregnancy test if appropriate.	Blood pressure check weekly for first month and after every dose increase, then every 1–3 mo CBC, serum Cr, BUN, LFT, lipids, magnesium potassium, uric acid every 2 wk for first month, then monthly. Interval pregnancy test if appropriate.	2–5 mg/kg/d	Rescue medication for all types of psoriasis (rapid onset)	Headache, nausea, cytopenias, renal toxicity, hypertension, elevated potassium, hyperlipidemia, serious infection (rare). NMSC with long-term chronic use.	Pill and liquid suspension	Do not recommend for patients with history of PUVA treatment or concurrent phototherapy given risk of NMSC Do not administer live virus vaccines while on cyclosporine Avoid use in patients with history of kidney disease or high blood pressure No more than 1 y of continuous use
Methotrexate	CBC/diff, renal function, LFT, PPD or quant gold TB test. Hepatitis A, B, C, HIV for at risk patients. Pregnancy test if appropriate.	CBC 5–6 d after 1st dose, then CBC, renal function, LFT monthly for first 3–6 mo, after dose increase, then every 6 mo while on stable dose Annual TB test for at risk patients. Interval pregnancy test if appropriate.	0.2–0.7 mg/kg/wk PO or SQ, max dose 25 mg/wk Folic acid 1 mg q daily	All types of psoriasis Prevention of anti-drug antibody formation on biologics	GI upset, fatigue, bone marrow suppression, hepatotoxicity, pulmonary toxicity, effects on mood.	Pill, liquid suspension, and solution for injection	Cannot be given with medications that interfere with folic acid metabolic pathway, such as trimethoprim-sulfamethoxazole. Avoid use in patients with history of liver disease, and adjust dose and use with caution in those with a history of kidney disease

Abbreviations: BUN, blood urea nitrogen; CBC, complete blood count; CBC/diff, complete blood count with differential; Cr, creatinine; HIV, human immunodeficiency virus; LFT, liver function tests; NB-UVB, narrow band UVB phototherapy; NMSC, non-melanoma skin cancer; PO, by mouth; PPD, protein derivative test; Quant Gold, Quantiferon gold; SQ, subcutaneous; TB,tuberculosis; UA-urinalysis.

*Individualize lab monitoring orders and frequency to the clinical context.

Adapted from Cordoro, KM, Kittler, NW, Lalor, L, Holland K, Tollefson, M., Psoriasis, *Pediatric Dermatology*, Schachner, LA and Hansen, RC, 4th edition, Elsevier and AAD NPF Pediatric Psoriasis Guidelines.

Table 4
Mechanism of action, dosing, monitoring, and side effects of targeted systemic treatment of psoriasis

Class	Drug	Mechanism of Action	Baseline Labs	Monitoring	Dosing and Frequency	Common Adverse Effects	Comments
Anti-TNFα	Etanercept	Soluble fusion protein of TNFα- receptor and Fc portion of human IgG	PPD or Quant Gold, Hep B,C, and HIV[a]	Yearly TB test with PPD or Quant Gold	≥ 63 kg, ~0.8 mg/kg/weekly SQ If > 63 kg, 50 mg	Injection site reaction, upper respiratory tract infection, headache, dizziness, sore throat, cough, abdominal pain, rhinitis	Update patient and household contact vaccinations prior to starting treatment. Avoid live and attenuated vaccines. Avoid in patients with history of MS or strong family history of MS.
	Infliximab	Chimeric monoclonal IgG antibody targeted TNFα	PPD or Quant Gold, Hep B,C, and HIV[a]	Yearly TB test with PPD or Quant Gold	IV 3.3–5 mg/kg at weeks 0,2,6, and then every 7–8 wk	Infusion reaction, upper respiratory tract infection, headache, rash, cough, abdominal pain	
	Adalimumab	Fully humanized monoclonal IgG antibody targeting TNFα	PPD or Quant Gold, Hep B,C, and HIV[a]	Yearly TB test with PPD or Quant Gold	~ 24 mg/m^2 or 0.8 mg/kg SQ (maximum 40 mg) weekly for the first 2 wk then every 2 wk	Injection site reaction, upper respiratory tract infection, abdominal pain, nausea, headache, rash, sinusitis, urinary tract infection.	
IL-17 inhibitors	Secukinumab	Fully human IgG1 monoclonal antibody that selectively binds IL-17A	PPD or Quant Gold,[b] Hep B,C, and HIV[a]	Yearly TB test with PPD or Quant Gold	≥50 kg, 150 mg SQ at week 0, 1, 2, 3, 4, then every 4 wk >25 to <50 kg 75 mg SQ at week 0, 1, 2, 3, 4, then every 4 wk <25 kg 75 mg SQ at week 0, 1, 2, 3, 4, then every 4 wk	Injection site reaction, nasopharyngitis, headache and pharyngitis, rhinitis	Avoid use in patients with personal history and use with caution in patient with family history of IBD Update patient and household contact vaccinations prior to starting treatment. Avoid live and attenuated vaccines.
	Ixekizumab	Humanized IgG monoclonal antibody that selectively binds IL-17A	PPD or Quant Gold,[b] Hep B,C, and HIV[a]	Yearly TB test with PPD or Quant Gold	> 50 kg, 160 mg SQ at Week 0, followed by 80 mg every 4 wk. >25–50 kg, 80 mg SQ at Week 0, followed by 40 mg every 4 wk. < 25 kg, 40 mg SQ at Week 0, followed by 20 mg every 4 wk.	Upper respiratory tract infection, nasopharyngitis, conjunctivitis, tonsilitis, oral candidiasis	

(*continued on next page*)

Table 4
(continued)

Class	Drug	Mechanism of Action	Baseline Labs	Monitoring	Dosing and Frequency	Common Adverse Effects	Comments
IL-12/23 inhibitor	Ustekinumab	Fully human monoclonal antibody targeting p40 subunit of IL-12 and IL-23	PPD or Quant Gold,[b] Hep B,C, and HIV[a]	Yearly TB test with PPD or Quant Gold	< 60 kg, 0.75 mg/kg SQ at weeks 0, 4 and then every 12 wk 60–100 kg, 45 mg, SQ at weeks 0, 4 and then every 12 wk > 100 kg, 90 mg SQ at weeks 0, 4 and then every 12 wk	Upper respiratory tract infection, headache, fatigue, redness at injection site, back pain.	Update patient and household contact vaccinations prior to starting treatment. Avoid live and attenuated vaccines.
PDE-4 inhibitor	Apremilast	Small molecule that blocks PDE4	None	None	> 20 kg, 20 mg BID PO[c] > 35 kg, 20–30 mg BID PO[c]	Nausea, headache, abdominal pain, nasopharyngitis, nausea, diarrhea	Depression associated with apremilast in adult trials. Phase 3 trials underway in children. Use with caution in pediatric patients with history of depression.

Abbreviations: BID, twice daily; CD, Crohn's Disease; IBD, inflammatory bowel disease; JIA, juvenile idiopathic arthritis; Quant Gold, Quantiferon gold; SQ, subcutaneous; TB, tuberculosis; UC, ulcerative colitis.

[a] Per manufacturer instructions, TB infection should be ruled out prior to starting medication. However, HIV, Hepatitis B, and hepatitis C screening should be carried out pending individual risk factors of patient. Per FDA regulations only.

[b] Per manufacturer instructions, TB infection should be ruled out prior to starting medication. However, it is unclear if TB testing is needed in biologic classes other than Anti-TNFα inhibitors.

[c] Dosing based on phase 2 clinical trial data for the approval of apremilast in children 6 y and older.

Adapted from Cordoro, KM, Kittler, NW, Lalor, L, Holland K, Tollefson, M., Psoriasis, *Pediatric Dermatology*, Schachner, LA and Hansen, RC, 4th edition, Elsevier and AAD NPF Pediatric Psoriasis Guidelines.

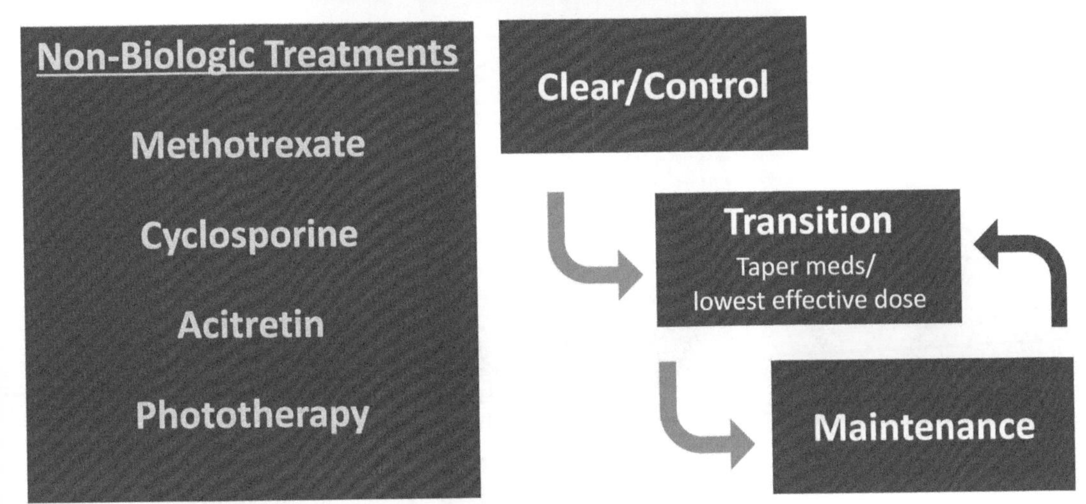

Fig. 3. 3 phases of therapy for non-biologic treatment.

of pustular and guttate psoriasis, as well as palmoplantar psoriasis. It is generally well tolerated and the most common side effects are mucocutaneous including xerosis, cheilitis, and granulation.[72] It can cause transaminitis and hypertriglyceridemia that are reversible upon dose reduction or cessation. Acitretin can be combined with NB-UVB, cyclosporine or MTX. Importantly, acitretin is not hepatotoxic,[73] like methotrexate. It has been reported to reduce methotrexate induced liver fibrosis when used in conjunction with methotrexate.[74]

METHOTREXATE

Illustrative Case in an Infant, a Continuation: Case 2b

The patient described above is now 14 months old. He has had psoriasis since age 3 months of age, initially controlled with, and now maintained on, low dose acitretin at a dose of 0.3 mg/kg every other day. He returns to your office for a flare of his psoriasis (**Fig. 5**). Given his severe flare, options for control include increasing the dose of acitretin, adding cyclosporine, methotrexate or a biologic. Sharing the decision with mom, it was decided to add methotrexate at a dosage of 0.3 mg/kg/wk. He achieves clearance in 8 weeks, the methotrexate is ultimately tapered, and he remains in remission on acitretin 0.3 mg/kg three times weekly (see **Fig. 5**).

Methotrexate is the most commonly prescribed systemic medication for pediatric patients with psoriasis worldwide.[75] It can be used for all subtypes of psoriasis and can help prevent formation of anti-drug antibodies when used concurrently with TNFα inhibitors.[76] Methotrexate has a slower onset but can achieve sustained remission. In a study evaluating the safety and efficacy of methotrexate for the treatment of psoriasis in pediatric patients, PASI75 was achieved in 4.3% and 33.3% of patients at week 12 and 24 after starting methotrexate. However, 40% of patients[77] reached PASI 75 at week 36.[77] In a retrospective study of children with psoriasis who were treated with methotrexate, when remission was achieved, it lasted up to 3 years.[78] Regarding the case above, once he achieves control, the methotrexate and then acitretin would ideally be weaned, and the patient maintained on topicals. Should his psoriasis flare again, a biologic would be considered to reduce total exposure to immunosuppressant agents at this age. In fact, this child did go on to have another severe pustular flare requiring admission (see continuation of case below in IL-17 Inhibitor section).

CYCLOSPORINE

Illustrative Case: Case 3

An 18 years old female with history of plaque psoriasis presents to your office with a severe guttate flare a few months before she is scheduled to depart for college (**Fig. 6**). Pharyngeal culture grows β-hemolytic streptococcus. She is otherwise healthy and baseline blood pressure and labs are normal. She takes oral contraceptive pills and no other medications. She is started on

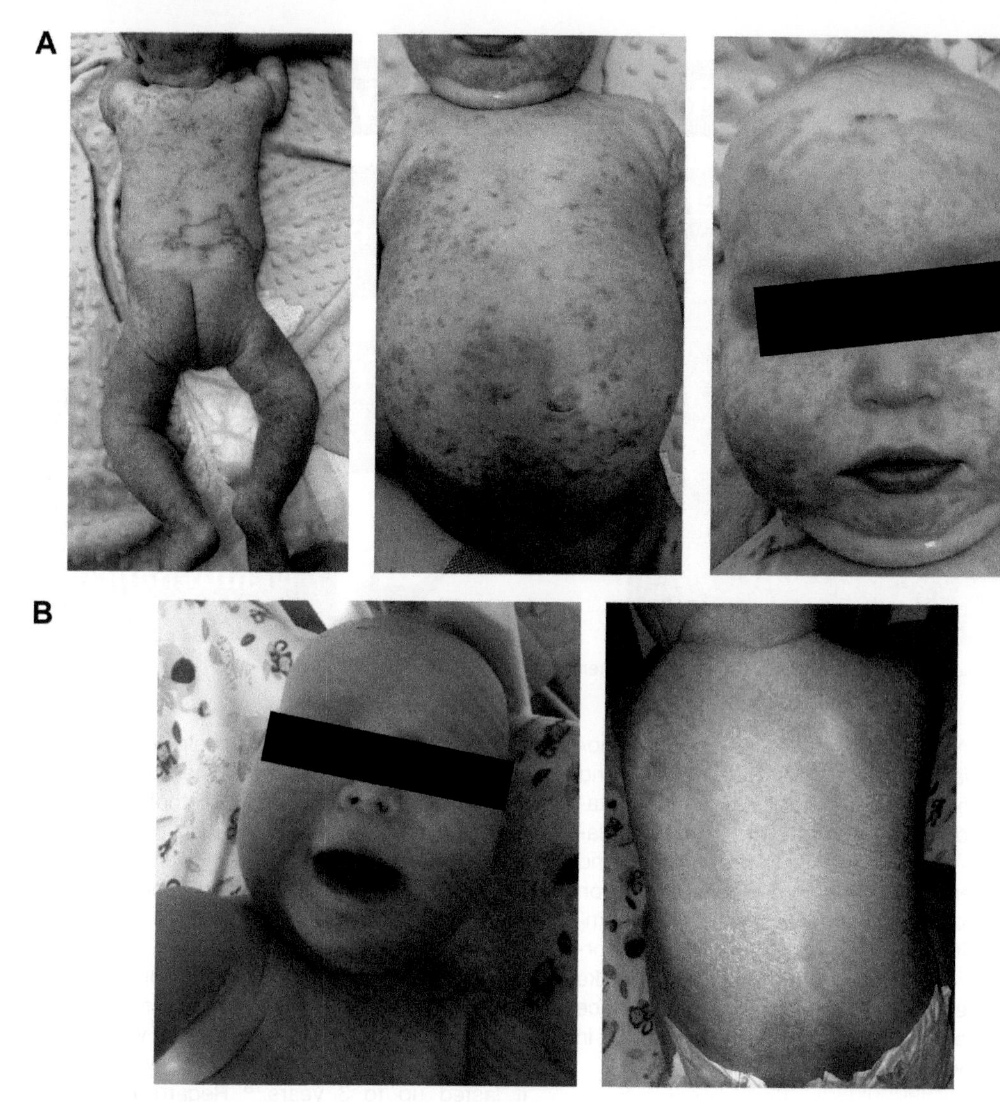

Fig. 4. Illustrative Case 2. An 8-month-old infant with severe psoriasis starting at 3 months of age. (*A*) On exam he is found to have psoriasis involving ~75% BSA with mixed morphology including annular plaques, diffuse scaly pink papules, and scattered pustules. (*B*) After 5 weeks of acitretin, his skin is nearly clear.

culture-directed antibiotics and cyclosporine 3 mg/kg/d for its rapid onset of action. After 2 months, she has a partial response but is otherwise tolerating cyclosporine well. Her dosage is increased to 5 mg/kg/d and her psoriasis nearly clears. After 8 months, she is completely clear and tapered off cyclosporine (see **Fig. 6**).

Cyclosporine is a powerful treatment option with a rapid onset that can be utilized as a rescue medication to gain control of psoriasis. It may be used in patients of all ages. Very young patients can tolerate higher starting doses of 5 mg/kg/d or more because of the pharmacokinetics of the drug in this age group, while adolescents and young adults are often started on lower doses and escalated as needed. Once clear, cyclosporine should be tapered to the lowest effective dose and then discontinued. A significant subset will relapse after discontinuation and therefore patients may need to transition to a different systemic or biologic medication for long-term maintenance. Due to associated long-term side effects, it is recommended that cyclosporine not be used continuously for more than 1 year.

"NEW AND NOVEL"

Targeted Therapies

The "new and novel" treatments have been developed more recently and selectively target components of the psoriasis inflammatory cascade. These include monoclonal antibodies against TNFα, IL-12/23, IL-23 and IL-17, and the small molecule phosphodiesterase 4 (PDE-4) inhibitor, apremilast (see **Table 4**). These treatments are overall more

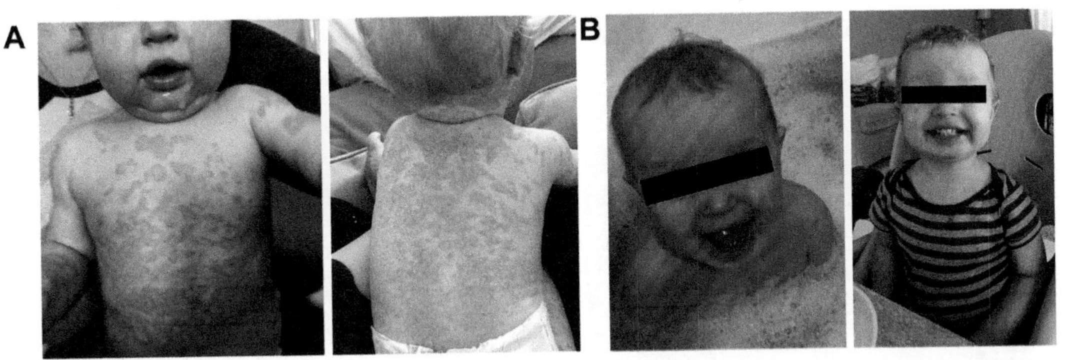

Fig. 5. Illustrative Case 2b. (*A*) now 14-month old infant with severe psoriasis starting at 3 months of age is now flaring on acitretin. Methotrexate is added to acitretin and is tapered after clearance is achieved. (*B*) He remains clear on acitretin at 24 months of age.

convenient when compared to conventional systemic treatments, more effective in practice and per the scant comparative data available, and the safety data is reassuring. If a patient is transitioning to a biologic from a conventional systemic for lack of efficacy, there is no overlap needed. Overlap is reasonable in patients with good efficacy on a systemic who are transitioning to a biologic for long-term maintenance. No washout period is necessary when transitioning from one biologic to another. Biologics require far less lab monitoring resulting in less missed school for patients and less missed work and lost productivity for caretakers. However, these therapies can be significantly more expensive compared to traditional systemic therapies. The expectation with the use of biologics is that patients will experience near or complete clearance and then continue the agent as maintenance. There are no pediatric data to guide treatment duration and therefore endpoint of therapy is a challenging issue to navigate in practice. Long-term continuous use beyond a reasonable period of remission is an unrealistic and probably unnecessary goal for many pediatric patients. Clinical data in adults suggests that intermittent treatment with biologics may be an effective, safe and well-tolerated option for certain patients. Despite their immunogenicity which induces formation of neutralizing antibodies, most biologic agents except for the mouse/human chimer infliximab maintained their efficacy and safety with intermittent use.[79]

TNFα INHIBITORS

Illustrative Case: Case 4

8 years old patient presents with an acute episode of severe generalized pustular psoriasis. The psoriasis failed to respond to high dose cyclosporine and the patient had to be admitted due to extent and systemic symptoms. Patient was started on infliximab and experienced dramatic improvement within 48 hours of initial infusion (**Fig. 7**). This patient had several previous episodes of pustular psoriasis, and responded to and then flared through trials of each of the conventional systemics alone and in combination, as well as the anti- TNFα agents. He was ultimately determined to have DITRA on genetic testing, responded to and then broke through several biologics, and is now in stable long-term remission on secukinumab. The details of his case are continued below, and have been published.[53]

Etanercept

Etanercept was the first biologic studied and ultimately approved for use by the FDA in 2016 for pediatric psoriasis patients aged 4 and older. It has a long term track record of good efficacy and excellent safety.[80–82] It is an excellent choice for younger patients given its approval to age 4, though the weekly injection schedule poses barriers for many children.

Adalimumab

Adalimumab is an anti TNFα agent not yet FDA approved for the treatment of pediatric psoriasis in the US, but is FDA approved for the treatment of JIA in children ages 2 and older, and for Crohn's in children ages 6 and older. Adalimumab is approved by the European Medical Agency for the treatment of psoriasis in children 4 years and older. Adalimumab showed good efficacy and safety versus methotrexate in children and adolescents with severe chronic plaque psoriasis in a randomized, double-blind, phase 3 trial.[81] It is particularly attractive choice for patients with overlap of hidradenitis suppurativa, as it is approved for this indication in pediatric patients aged 12 years and older.[83]

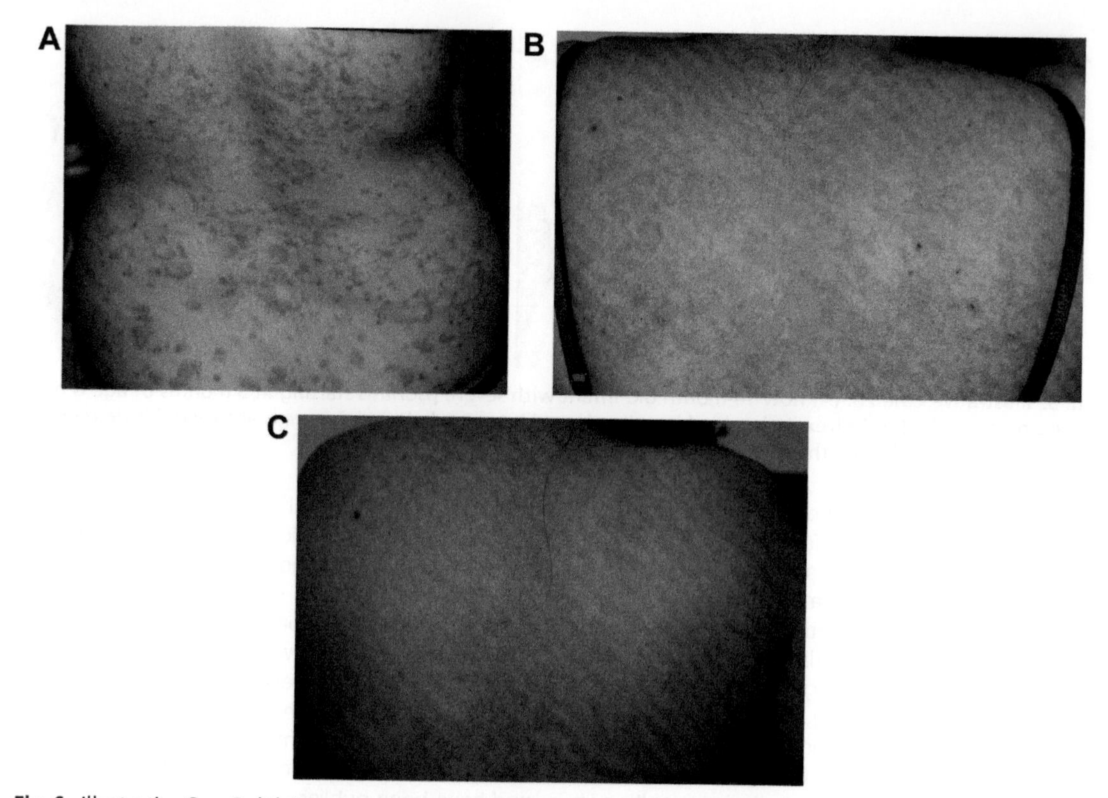

Fig. 6. Illustrative Case 3. (*A*) 18-year-old female with history of plaque psoriasis with a severe guttate flare due to β-hemolytic streptococcus. (*B*) She has some improvement after 1 month of cyclosporine 3 mg/kg/d. (*C*) Her skin is nearly clear after 3 months of cyclosporine 5 mg/kg/d.

Infliximab

Infliximab is an anti TNFα medication that is not FDA approved for the treatment of pediatric psoriasis, but is FDA approved for the treatment of ulcerative colitis (UC) and CD in children 6 years and older. In adults, it has been shown to have overall good safety and efficacy data for the treatment of psoriasis. It is administered via intravenous infusion, and its onset can be very rapid within hours to days, making it an excellent choice for patients needing immediate control as illustrated in the case above. The requirement for infusions may serve as a barrier to access, but also helps with adherence as this is a facility-administered treatment. The molecule is a mouse/human chimer, and development of antibodies may reduce efficacy and result in infusion reactions over time.[84]

IL-12/23 INHIBITOR
Illustrative Cases

Young child: case 5

A 6 years old presents for rapid progression of psoriasis. Family history is notable for mother with psoriasis who is currently on a TNFα inhibitor. On exam, the patient has scattered plaque psoriasis on the extremities and throughout most of the scalp with extension onto the forehead (**Fig. 8**). Given mom's negative experiences living with psoriasis, the child's severe disease and her interest in minimizing frequency of injections, a shared decision is made to start ustekinumab. The family appreciated knowing this agent is approved to age 6 and has excellent efficacy and safety data for use in children. Moreover, the fact that this medication only requires an injection every 3 months is very appealing for both the patient and her mother. At follow-up just a few months later, she has nearly complete clearance. She and her mother are very pleased with her results.

Adolescent: a Continuation of Cyclosporine Case: Case 3b

A 19 years old female with history of plaque psoriasis presents for follow-up. She previously achieved clearance of a severe guttate flare with cyclosporine and has been clear for the last 7 months. However, she recently noticed recurrence of psoriatic plaques on the trunk and extremities (**Fig. 9**). She has dealt with psoriasis on

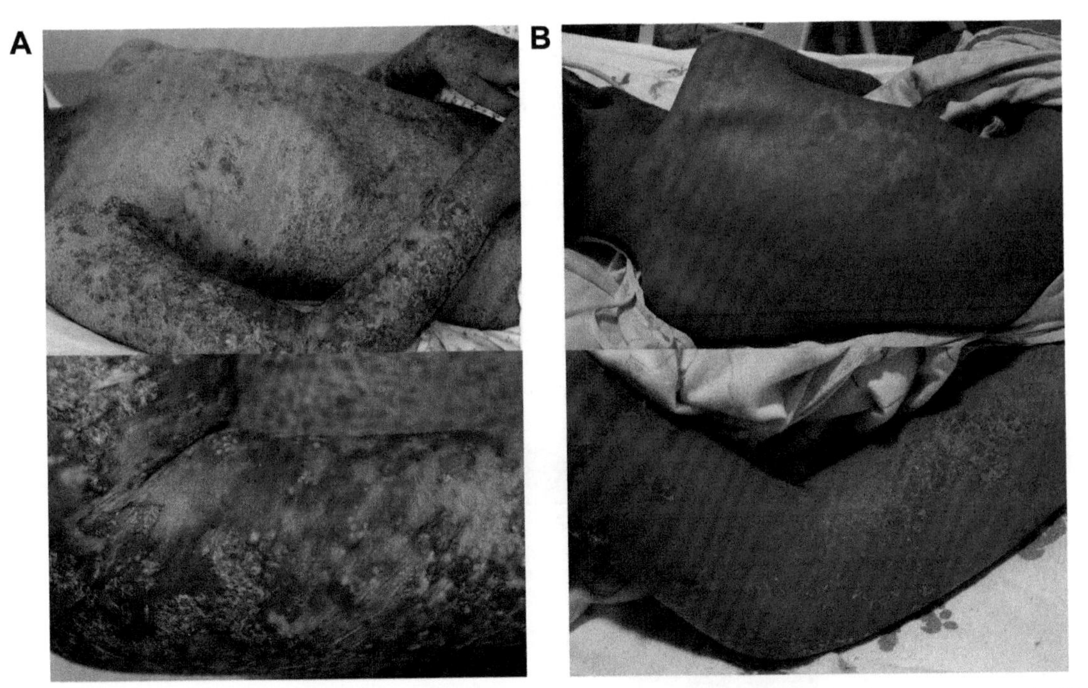

Fig. 7. Illustrative case 4. (*A*) 8-year-old male with an acute episode of severe generalized pustular psoriasis. (*B*) He is started on infliximab and has had dramatic improvement within 48 hours of initial infusion. He is ultimately determined to have DITRA, and achieves long-term remission on secukinumab.

and off for the last 10 years, has just started college, and would like a long-term option. She is interested in trying a new medication but is hesitant to give herself an injection. A decision is made to start apremilast; however, insurance denies this medication despite multiple appeals. Ustekinumab is prescribed given its quarterly injection schedule which the patient can manage while in college. After the first 2 injections (initial dose and loading dose 1 month later), her psoriasis clears and has remained clear for 3 years on continuous therapy. She has had no adverse effects.

CARD-14 associated papulosquamous eruption (CAPE): case 6

An adolescent male with lifelong psoriasis/PRP overlap was recently found to have a mutation in the *CARD14* gene. His condition had failed to respond to or had modest improvement with methotrexate, acitretin and TNFα inhibition in the past. Ustekinumab therapy resulted in dramatic improvement in his erythroderma, scale, itch and quality of life (**Fig. 10**). He has been on therapy for 3 years now with sustained efficacy. His case is part of a series detailing the clinical phenotype, genotype and therapy for CAPE.[65]

Ustekinumab

Ustekinumab is an IL-12/23 inhibitor and is approved to treat moderate to severe plaque psoriasis in children ages 6 years and older. It has been shown to have an overall high efficacy and good safety profile. Results of the CADMUS phase 3 trial, which included children ages 12 to 17 years old, demonstrated a PASI 75 of at least 78.4% at week 12.[85] Similarly, results of the CADMUS Jr phase 3 trial, which included children ages 6 to 12 years old, demonstrated PASI 75 in 85% of patients receiving ustekinumab at week 12.[86] Ustekinumab has the least frequent and thus most favorable maintenance injection schedule (once every 12 weeks). As discussed above, ustekinumab has emerged as the current treatment of choice for patients with *CARD 14* mediated psoriasis.[67]

IL-17 INHIBITORS

Illustrative Case: Continuation of Generalized Pustular Psoriasis in an Adolescent: Case 4b

An adolescent male with lifelong history of intermittent episodes of generalized pustular psoriasis is admitted for a severe exacerbation. His skin has failed to respond to, or broken through, multiple treatments including methotrexate, cyclosporine, acitretin, adalimumab, and ustekinumab. He had rapid response to infliximab during a prior admission for a febrile generalized pustular flare, and was continued as an outpatient on adalimumab due to lack of proximity to an infusion center which precluded ongoing infliximab therapy. On this

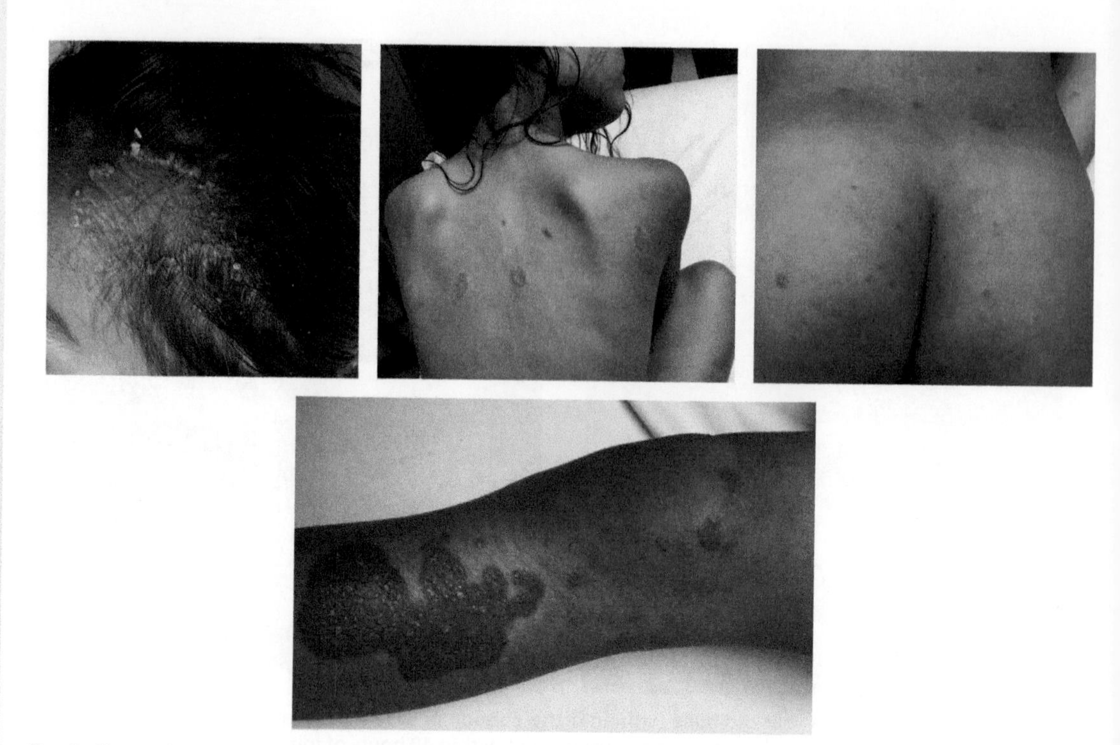

Fig. 8. Illustrative case 5. A 6 year old female presents for rapid progression of psoriasis. On exam, she is found to have scattered plaque psoriasis on the extremities and throughout most of the scalp with extension onto the forehead. A decision is made to start ustekinumab; at follow up 2 months later she has nearly complete clearance.

admission, however, treatment with intravenous infliximab resulted in a severe infusion reaction. Anakinra was trialed during admission for suspected DITRA, but his skin and overall clinical status deteriorated on this therapy. Blood was drawn for genomics and tissue was biopsied for immune phenotyping. Flow cytometry of biopsied lesional skin revealed markedly high production of IL-17A from CD4+ T cells. Secukinumab was started to target the elevated IL-17. The patient had a rapid and robust clinical and laboratory response, with defervescence within 12 hours, cessation of new pustule formation within 24 hours, and was discharged after 48 hours. His skin was nearly clear at follow-up 3 days after discharge. Genetic analysis later confirmed the presence of a mutation in the *IL36RN* gene and thus a diagnosis of DITRA. He has remained in long-term (greater than 3 years) remission on secukinumab without adverse effects.

Severe Mixed Morphology Psoriasis in a Toddler, a Continuation: Case 2c

This child is now 3 years old. His previously severe plaque/pustular psoriasis has been maintained on intermittent, low dose acitretin (0.3 mg/kg 3 times per week) since the age of 14 months. At last office visit 6 months ago, his skin was 100% clear. Mom called 10 days ago stating that he abruptly developed rapidly progressing widespread plaques and pustules. At that time, cyclosporine 5 mg/kg/d was added, but his condition continued to deteriorate. He was admitted to our hospital due to the extent of his condition, though he remained systemically well other than mild malaise and fatigue despite dramatic skin involvement (**Fig. 11**). Treatment considerations at that point were limited to rapid onset targeted therapy, and we preferred an IL-17 inhibitor in this case. Insurance would only cover etanercept, which was started as an inpatient. He also received wet wrap therapy with topical corticosteroids (0.1% triamcinolone ointment body and hydrocortisone 2.5% ointment face and anogenital area) while in-house, and his condition began to improve. He was discharged on low dose acitretin, cyclosporine, and weekly etanercept. Three weeks later, he developed widespread pustules. Insurance was petitioned to cover the anti-IL-17 agent ixekizumab, which ultimately was approved, and his psoriasis has been nearly clear for 6 months. Cyclosporine then acitretin were weaned off. On ixekizumab monotherapy, he continues to have occasional localized pustular episodes temporally associated with mild viral upper respiratory infections, but has

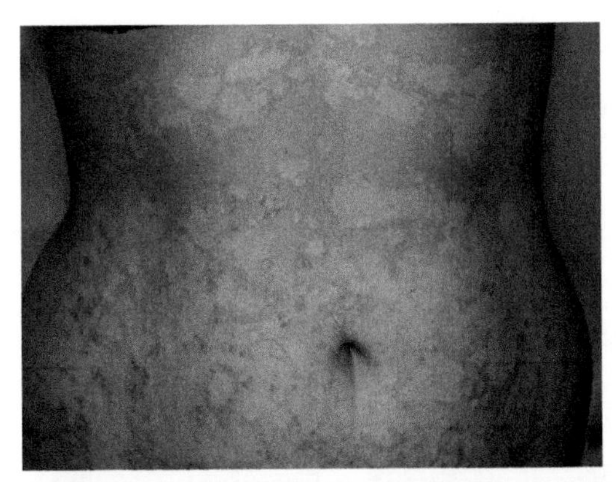

Fig. 9. Illustrative Case 3b. (*A*) A now 19-year-old female with history of plaque psoriasis previously cleared on cyclosporine is now flaring 7 months after discontinuing cyclosporine. On exam she is found to have recurrent psoriatic plaques on the trunk and extremities.

not had generalized pustular psoriasis since starting ixekizumab. We are re-interrogating his genome to confirm absence of relevant mutations.

Secukinumab and Ixekizumab

IL-17 inhibitors selectively target IL-17 in the psoriasis inflammatory cascade. While all may be called upon to treat pediatric psoriasis, only ixekizumab and secukinumab are currently FDA-approved for children aged 6 and older with moderate to severe plaque psoriasis. Ixekizumab was the first to be approved after studies showed rapid and statistically significant improvements over placebo in skin involvement, itch and health-related quality of life, which persisted through 48 weeks of treatment in pediatric patients aged 6 to 18 years with moderate-to-severe plaque psoriasis.[87] Secukinumab was most recently approved for the treatment of moderate to severe plaque psoriasis in children ages 6 and older based on trial data demonstrating excellent safety and efficacy. Both high and low dose secukinumab were superior to placebo and etanercept.[88]

IL-17 inhibitors are ideally avoided in patients with inflammatory bowel disease (IBD) and used with caution in those with a strong family history of IBD as IL17 inhibitors may exacerbate the condition.[68]

TARGETED THERAPIES IN THE PIPELINE

Several targeted therapies are in clinical trials for pediatric psoriasis, including ongoing phase 3 trials for certolizumab (TNFα inhibitor), guselkumab (IL- 23 inhibitor), risankizumab (IL-23 inhibitor), brodalumab (IL- 17 inhibitor), and apremilast (PDE-4 inhibitor). These trials have the potential to significantly broaden the targeted treatment options available to pediatric patients by expanding the limited safety and efficacy data currently available. See **Table 2** for a summary of current trials.

PUTTING IT ALL TOGETHER: CASE 1 REVISITED

Taking both objective (BSA, functional limitations) and subjective (psychological impact) measures of severity together, it is very clear that this patient has severe psoriasis and needs rapid relief. A shared decision with family is made to start adalimumab given the family's familiarity with this medication. However, this is denied by his insurance. As an appeal is prepared, plans are made to start methotrexate and soak and seal therapy with triamcinolone 0.1% ointment. Baseline labs are notable for mildly elevated liver enzymes which are attributed to systemic inflammation. The patient is given a test dose of 5 mg of methotrexate followed by CBC 5 days later which is normal. Folate supplementation of 1 mg daily is

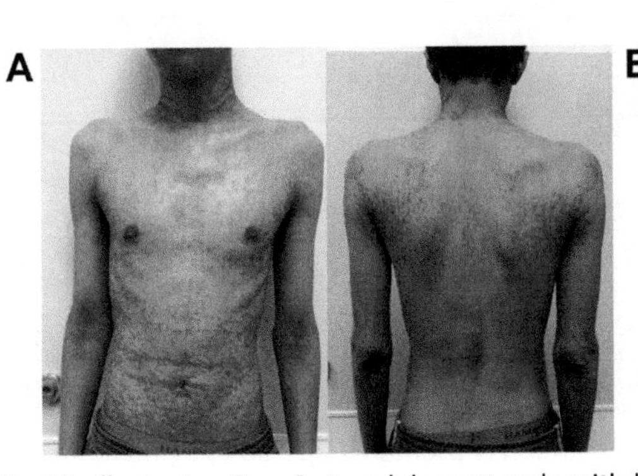

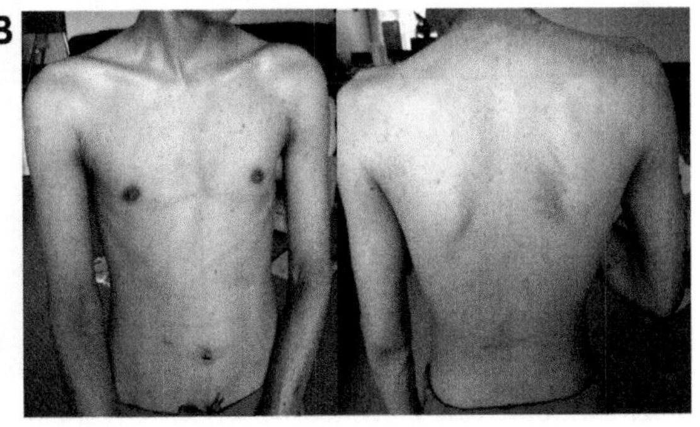

Fig. 10. Illustrative Case 6. An adolescent male with lifelong psoriasis/PRP overlap was recently found to have a mutation in the CARD14 gene. (*A*) On exam he is found to have a background of erythroderma with overlying scale. (*B*) Ustekinumab is started, and he has dramatic improvement in his erythroderma, scale, itch and quality of life.

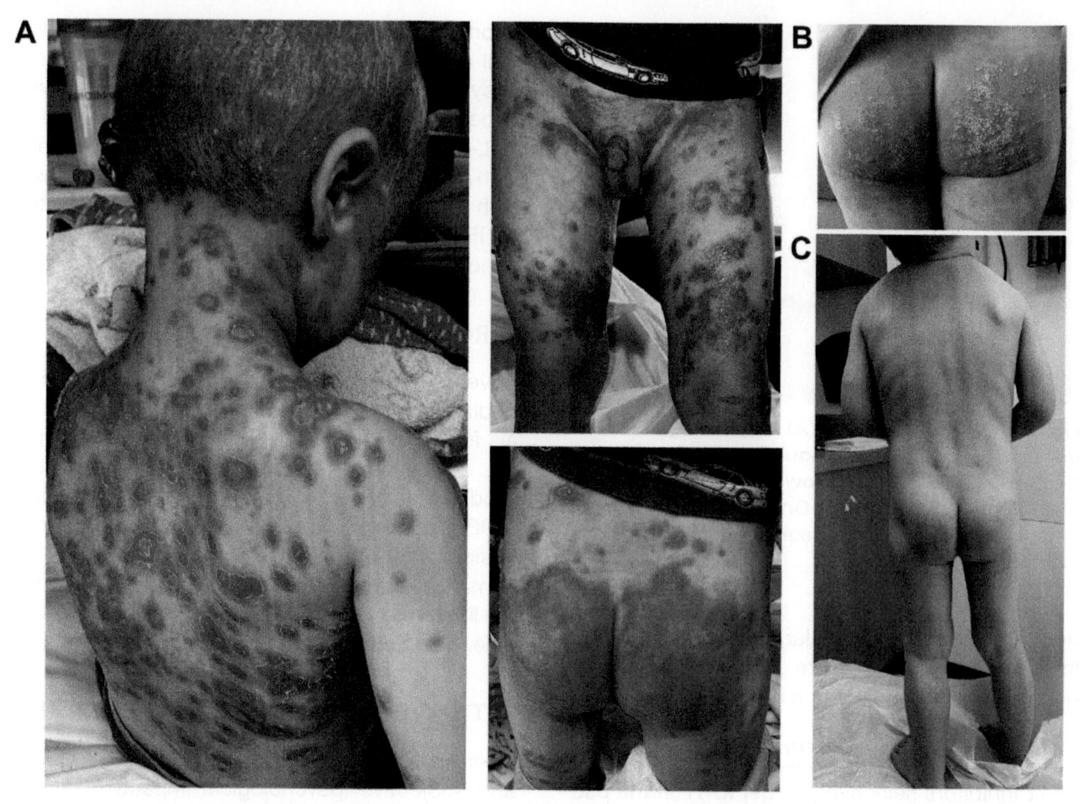

Fig. 11. Illustrative Case 2c. (*A*) A now 3-year-old male with severe psoriasis starting at 3 months of age is flaring again on acitretin with widespread plaques and pustules. Cyclosporine is added, but his condition continues to deteriorate, and he is admitted to the hospital. He is started on etanercept and is discharged on low dose acitretin, cyclosporine, and weekly etanercept. (*B*) Three weeks later, he starts to develop widespread pustules. Etanercept is stopped and ixekizumab initiated with near clearance of his skin (*C*) with near clearance of his skin.

prescribed. His MTX dose is escalated to 12.5 mg then 15 mg weekly (roughly 0.5 mg/kg/wk). Follow up liver enzymes normalized and CBC remains normal. Three weeks later, his skin has improved by 50% on methotrexate and soak and seal. Adalimumab is approved by his insurance. Though his trajectory is favorable, given the severity of his disease, its chronicity and impact beyond the skin,

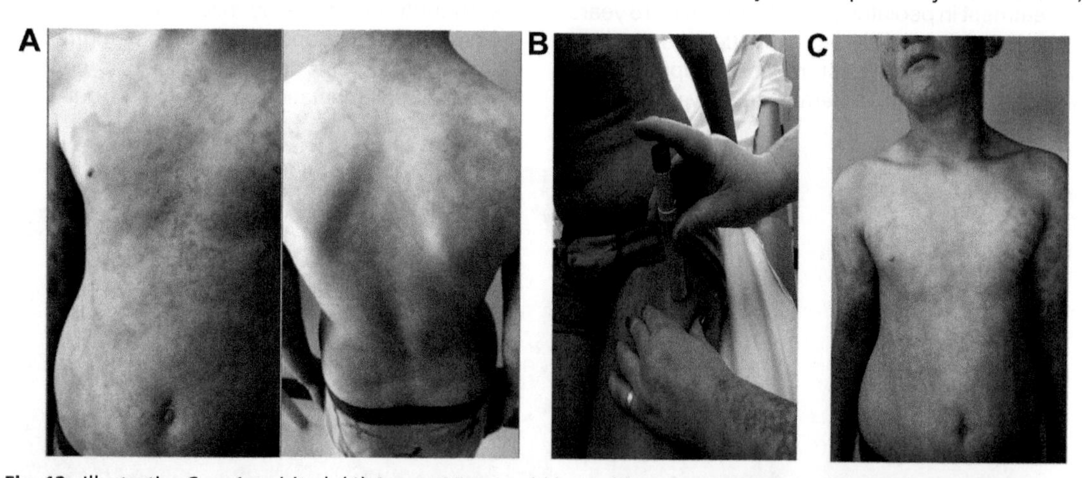

Fig. 12. Illustrative Case 1 revisited. (*A*) A now 10-year-old boy with severe psoriasis is s/p 3 doses of methotrexate. On exam he is found to have significant improvement, but continues to have plaques of the scalp, fac, trunk, extremities, genitals, palms and soles. (*B*) The decision is made to add adalimumab, which is administered in the office by the patient's mother. (*C*) The patient is now s/p 2 months of adalimumab in addition to methotrexate. On exam, his skin is almost completely clear.

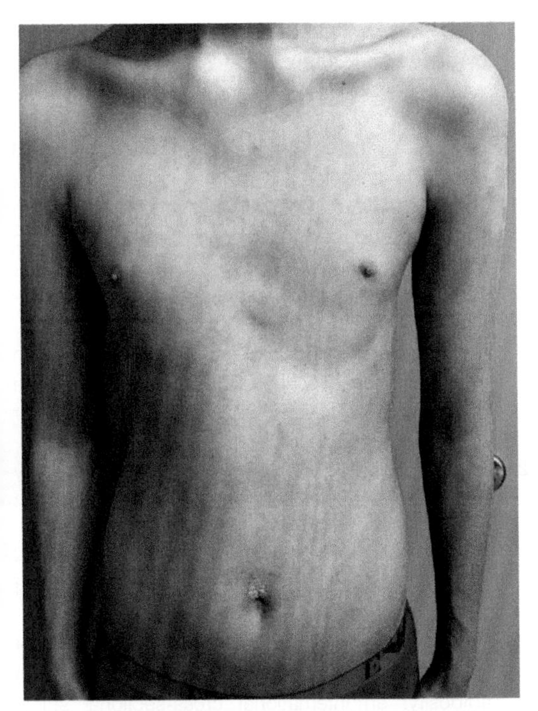

Fig. 13. Illustrative Case 1 revisited. The patient is now 15 years and has nearly completely clear skin on adalimumab. He is otherwise doing well and thriving.

and family history of psoriasis, the decision is made to proceed with adalimumab and the first dose is administered in the office by his mother, with supervision (**Fig. 12**).

At follow-up 2 months later, his skin is almost completely clear (see **Fig. 12**). Methotrexate is tapered to 5 mg weekly to help block the formation of anti-drug antibodies, and topical therapy is discontinued. He is referred to a therapist for severe anxiety, depression, and anger.

At his most recent follow-up 4 years after this severe flare and initiation of systemic therapy, he is a happy, healthy, well-adjusted 15 years old. His psoriasis is clear except for a persistent small plaque on the ankle (**Fig. 13**). He has had no side effects of therapy and is participating in activities with peers. He is thriving on adalimumab and MTX 5 mg q week, and has been psychologically well enough to stop sessions with his therapist. The endpoint of this child's therapy is unclear, and we will continue to work with him to determine whether a trial period off therapy makes sense for him.

SUMMARY AND DISCUSSION

Treating and managing pediatric patients with moderate to severe psoriasis can be challenging. The decision to start a systemic therapy must account for several patient and drug-related factors. With the exception of treating DIRA, DITRA or CAPE, or psoriasis in patients with IBD or other contraindications to certain therapies, all options should be equally considered and selection should reflect a tailored approach for each patient's individual needs and family preferences. "Tried and true" therapies including acitretin, methotrexate and cyclosporine are supported by decades of use demonstrating safety and efficacy. These medicines are cost effective when compared to targeted treatments and can be started and stopped relatively easily. However, frequent lab monitoring is often required. "New and novel" treatments include monoclonal antibodies against TNFα, IL-12/23, IL-23 and IL-17 and the small molecule phosphodiesterase 4 (PDE-4) inhibitor, apremilast. These medications have overall high efficacy, favorable safety, and require very little lab monitoring, but downsides are the need for injections, unclear endpoint of therapy, and high cost which poses an access barrier. Importantly, pediatric psoriasis is a condition under intense study and children now benefit from a treatment tool box filled with more therapeutic options than ever before.

DISCLOSURE

The authors have no disclosures, conflicts of interest, or funding sources to declare.

REFERENCES

1. Vogel SA, Yentzer B, Davis SA, et al. Trends in pediatric psoriasis outpatient health care delivery in the United States. Arch Dermatol 2012;148(1):66–71.
2. Cordoro KM, Hitraya-Low M, Taravati K, et al. Skin-infiltrating, interleukin-22-producing T cells differentiate pediatric psoriasis from adult psoriasis. J Am Acad Dermatol 2017;77(3):417–24.
3. Huppler AR, Bishu S, Gaffen SL. Mucocutaneous candidiasis: the IL-17 pathway and implications for targeted immunotherapy. Arthritis Res Ther 2012;14(4):217.
4. Saunte DM, Mrowietz U, Puig L, et al. Candida infections in patients with psoriasis and psoriatic arthritis treated with interleukin-17 inhibitors and their practical management. Br J Dermatol 2017;177(1):47–62.
5. Salek MS, Jung S, Brincat-Ruffini LA, et al. Clinical experience and psychometric properties of the Children's Dermatology Life Quality Index (CDLQI), 1995-2012. Br J Dermatol 2013;169(4):734–59.
6. DuBois DL, Bull CA, Sherman MD, et al. Self-esteem and adjustment in early adolescence: a social-

contextual perspective. J Youth Adolescence 1998;27(5):557–83.
7. MacPhee AR, Andrews JJ. Risk factors for depression in early adolescence. Adolescence 2006;41(163):435–66.
8. Rosenstrom T, Jokela M, Hintsanen M, et al. Body-image dissatisfaction is strongly associated with chronic dysphoria. J Affect Disord 2013;150(2):253–60.
9. Provini LE, Omandac VT, Bahrani E, et al. Cutaneous body image: a window into the adolescent experience of dermatologic disease. Pediatr Dermatol 2021;00:1–8.
10. Mercy K, Kwasny M, Cordoro KM, et al. Clinical manifestations of pediatric psoriasis: results of a multicenter study in the United States. Pediatr Dermatol 2013;30(4):424–8.
11. Naldi L, Peli L, Parazzini F, et al. Psoriasis study group of the italian group for epidemiological research in D. Family history of psoriasis, stressful life events, and recent infectious disease are risk factors for a first episode of acute guttate psoriasis: results of a case-control study. J Am Acad Dermatol 2001;44(3):433–8.
12. Raychaudhuri SP, Gross J. A comparative study of pediatric onset psoriasis with adult onset psoriasis. Pediatr Dermatol 2000;17(3):174–8.
13. Ko HC, Jwa SW, Song M, et al. Clinical course of guttate psoriasis: long-term follow-up study. J Dermatol 2010;37(10):894–9.
14. Beattie PE, Lewis-Jones MS. A comparative study of impairment of quality of life in children with skin disease and children with other chronic childhood diseases. Br J Dermatol 2006;155(1):145–51.
15. Varni JW, Globe DR, Gandra SR, et al. Health-related quality of life of pediatric patients with moderate to severe plaque psoriasis: comparisons to four common chronic diseases. Eur J Pediatr 2012;171(3):485–92.
16. de Jager ME, De Jong EM, Evers AW, et al. The burden of childhood psoriasis. Pediatr Dermatol 2011;28(6):736–7.
17. Randa H, Todberg T, Skov L, et al. Health-related quality of life in children and adolescents with psoriasis: a systematic review and meta-analysis. Acta Derm Venereol 2017;97(5):555–63.
18. Tollefson MM, Finnie DM, Schoch JJ, et al. Impact of childhood psoriasis on parents of affected children. J Am Acad Dermatol 2017;76(2):286–289 e285.
19. Kim GE, Seidler E, Kimball AB. Effect of age at diagnosis on chronic quality of life and long-term outcomes of individuals with psoriasis. Pediatr Dermatol 2015;32(5):656–62.
20. Osier E, Wang AS, Tollefson MM, et al. Pediatric psoriasis comorbidity screening guidelines. JAMA Dermatol 2017;153(7):698–704.
21. Kimball AB, Wu EQ, Guerin A, et al. Risks of developing psychiatric disorders in pediatric patients with psoriasis. J Am Acad Dermatol 2012;67(4):651–7.e1-2.
22. Kurd SK, Troxel AB, Crits-Christoph P, et al. The risk of depression, anxiety, and suicidality in patients with psoriasis: a population-based cohort study. Arch Dermatol 2010;146(8):891–5.
23. Singh S, Taylor C, Kornmehl H, et al. Psoriasis and suicidality: a systematic review and meta-analysis. J Am Acad Dermatol 2017;77(3):425–440 e422.
24. Todberg T, Egeberg A, Jensen P, et al. Psychiatric comorbidities in children and adolescents with psoriasis: a population-based cohort study. Br J Dermatol 2017;177(2):551–3.
25. Koo J, Marangell LB, Nakamura M, et al. Depression and suicidality in psoriasis: review of the literature including the cytokine theory of depression. J Eur Acad Dermatol Venereol 2017;31(12):1999–2009.
26. Becker L, Tom WL, Eshagh K, et al. Excess adiposity preceding pediatric psoriasis. JAMA Dermatol 2014;150(5):573–4.
27. Gutmark-Little I, Shah KN. Obesity and the metabolic syndrome in pediatric psoriasis. Clin Dermatol 2015;33(3):305–15.
28. Paller AS, Mercy K, Kwasny MJ, et al. Association of pediatric psoriasis severity with excess and central adiposity: an international cross-sectional study. JAMA Dermatol 2013;149(2):166–76.
29. Tollefson MM, Van Houten HK, Asante D, et al. Association of psoriasis with comorbidity development in children with psoriasis. JAMA Dermatol 2018;154(3):286–92.
30. Zhu KJ, He SM, Zhang C, et al. Relationship of the body mass index and childhood psoriasis in a Chinese Han population: a hospital-based study. J Dermatol 2012;39(2):181–3.
31. Bronckers IM, Paller AS, van Geel MJ, et al. Psoriasis in children and adolescents: diagnosis, management and comorbidities. Paediatr Drugs 2015;17(5):373–84.
32. Au SC, Goldminz AM, Loo DS, et al. Association between pediatric psoriasis and the metabolic syndrome. J Am Acad Dermatol 2012;66(6):1012–3.
33. Goldminz AM, Buzney CD, Kim N, et al. Prevalence of the metabolic syndrome in children with psoriatic disease. Pediatr Dermatol 2013;30(6):700–5.
34. Koebnick C, Black MH, Smith N, et al. The association of psoriasis and elevated blood lipids in overweight and obese children. J Pediatr 2011;159(4):577–83.
35. Boehncke WH, Boehncke S, Tobin AM, et al. The 'psoriatic march': a concept of how severe psoriasis may drive cardiovascular comorbidity. Exp Dermatol 2011;20(4):303–7.
36. Lan CC, Ko YC, Yu HS, et al. Methotrexate reduces the occurrence of cerebrovascular events among Taiwanese psoriatic patients: a nationwide population-based study. Acta Derm Venereol 2012;92(4):349–52.
37. Prodanovich S, Ma F, Taylor JR, et al. Methotrexate reduces incidence of vascular diseases in veterans

with psoriasis or rheumatoid arthritis. J Am Acad Dermatol 2005;52(2):262–7.
38. Wu JJ, Poon KY, Channual JC, et al. Association between tumor necrosis factor inhibitor therapy and myocardial infarction risk in patients with psoriasis. Arch Dermatol 2012;148(11):1244–50.
39. Menter A, Strober BE, Kaplan DH, et al. Joint AAD-NPF guidelines of care for the management and treatment of psoriasis with biologics. J Am Acad Dermatol 2019;80(4):1029–72.
40. Lewkowicz D, Gottlieb AB. Pediatric psoriasis and psoriatic arthritis. Dermatol Ther 2004;17(5):364–75.
41. Stoll ML, Punaro M. Psoriatic juvenile idiopathic arthritis: a tale of two subgroups. Curr Opin Rheumatol 2011;23(5):437–43.
42. Reddy S, Jia S, Geoffrey R, et al. An autoinflammatory disease due to homozygous deletion of the IL1RN locus. N Engl J Med 2009;360(23):2438–44.
43. Aksentijevich I, Masters SL, Ferguson PJ, et al. An autoinflammatory disease with deficiency of the interleukin-1-receptor antagonist. N Engl J Med 2009;360(23):2426–37.
44. Stenerson M, Dufendach K, Aksentijevich I, et al. The first reported case of compound heterozygous IL1RN mutations causing deficiency of the interleukin-1 receptor antagonist. Arthritis Rheum 2011;63(12):4018–22.
45. Minkis K, Aksentijevich I, Goldbach-Mansky R, et al. Interleukin 1 receptor antagonist deficiency presenting as infantile pustulosis mimicking infantile pustular psoriasis. Arch Dermatol 2012;148(6):747–52.
46. Jesus AA, Osman M, Silva CA, et al. A novel mutation of IL1RN in the deficiency of interleukin-1 receptor antagonist syndrome: description of two unrelated cases from Brazil. Arthritis Rheum 2011; 63(12):4007–17.
47. Marrakchi S, Guigue P, Renshaw BR, et al. Interleukin-36-receptor antagonist deficiency and generalized pustular psoriasis. N Engl J Med 2011;365(7): 620–8.
48. Onoufriadis A, Simpson MA, Pink AE, et al. Mutations in IL36RN/IL1F5 are associated with the severe episodic inflammatory skin disease known as generalized pustular psoriasis. Am J Hum Genet 2011; 89(3):432–7.
49. Pan J, Qiu L, Xiao T, et al. Juvenile generalized pustular psoriasis with IL36RN mutation treated with short-term infliximab. Dermatol Ther 2016;29(3): 164–7.
50. Rossi-Semerano L, Piram M, Chiaverini C, et al. First clinical description of an infant with interleukin-36-receptor antagonist deficiency successfully treated with anakinra. Pediatrics 2013;132(4):e1043–7.
51. Bonekamp N, Caorsi R, Viglizzo GM, et al. High-dose ustekinumab for severe childhood deficiency of interleukin-36 receptor antagonist (DITRA). Ann Rheum Dis 2018;77(8):1241–3.
52. Cherqaoui B Jr, Rossi-Semerano L, Piram M, et al. Standard dose of Ustekinumab for childhood-onset deficiency of interleukin-36 receptor antagonist. Ann Rheum Dis 2018;77(12):e88.
53. Cordoro KM, Ucmak D, Hitraya-Low M, et al. Response to Interleukin (IL)-17 Inhibition in an Adolescent With Severe Manifestations of IL-36 Receptor Antagonist Deficiency (DITRA). JAMA Dermatol 2017;153(1):106–8.
54. Ho PH, Tsai TF. Successful treatment of refractory juvenile generalized pustular psoriasis with secukinumab monotherapy: A case report and review of published work. J Dermatol 2018;45(11):1353–6.
55. Kostner K, Prelog M, Almanzar G, et al. Successful use of secukinumab in a 4-year-old patient with deficiency of interleukin-36 antagonist. Rheumatology (Oxford) 2018;57(5):936–8.
56. Molho-Pessach V, Alyan R, Gordon D, et al. Secukinumab for the treatment of deficiency of interleukin 36 receptor antagonist in an adolescent. JAMA Dermatol 2017;153(5):473–5.
57. Bachelez H, Choon SE, Marrakchi S, et al. Inhibition of the Interleukin-36 Pathway for the Treatment of Generalized Pustular Psoriasis. N Engl J Med 2019;380(10):981–3.
58. Jordan CT, Cao L, Roberson ED, et al. Rare and common variants in CARD14, encoding an epidermal regulator of NF-kappaB, in psoriasis. Am J Hum Genet 2012;90(5):796–808.
59. Ammar M, Jordan CT, Cao L, et al. CARD14 alterations in Tunisian patients with psoriasis and further characterization in European cohorts. Br J Dermatol 2016;174(2):330–7.
60. Berki DM, Liu L, Choon SE, et al. Activating CARD14 Mutations Are Associated with Generalized Pustular Psoriasis but Rarely Account for Familial Recurrence in Psoriasis Vulgaris. J Invest Dermatol 2015; 135(12):2964–70.
61. Coto-Segura P, Gonzalez-Fernandez D, Batalla A, et al. Common and rare CARD14 gene variants affect the antitumour necrosis factor response among patients with psoriasis. Br J Dermatol 2016; 175(1):134–41.
62. Fuchs-Telem D, Sarig O, van Steensel MA, et al. Familial pityriasis rubra pilaris is caused by mutations in CARD14. Am J Hum Genet 2012;91(1): 163–70.
63. Has C, Schwieger-Briel A, Schlipf N, et al. Target-sequence Capture and High Throughput Sequencing Identify a De novo CARD14 Mutation in an Infant with Erythrodermic Pityriasis Rubra Pilaris. Acta Derm Venereol 2016;96(7):989–90.
64. Jordan CT, Cao L, Roberson ED, et al. PSORS2 is due to mutations in CARD14. Am J Hum Genet 2012;90(5):784–95.
65. Sugiura K. The genetic background of generalized pustular psoriasis: IL36RN mutations and CARD14

gain-of-function variants. J Dermatol Sci 2014;74(3):187–92.
66. Takeichi T, Kobayashi A, Ogawa E, et al. Autosomal dominant familial generalized pustular psoriasis caused by a CARD14 mutation. Br J Dermatol 2017;177(4):e133–5.
67. Craiglow BG, Boyden LM, Hu R, et al. CARD14-associated papulosquamous eruption: a spectrum including features of psoriasis and pityriasis rubra pilaris. J Am Acad Dermatol 2018;79(3):487–94.
68. Hohenberger M, Cardwell LA, Oussedik E, et al. Interleukin-17 inhibition: role in psoriasis and inflammatory bowel disease. J Dermatolog Treat 2018;29(1):13–8.
69. Seccombe E, Wynne MD, Clancy C, et al. A retrospective review of phototherapy in children, at a tertiary paediatric dermatology unit. Photodermatol Photoimmunol Photomed 2021;37(1):34–8.
70. Kopp T, Karlhofer F, Szepfalusi Z, et al. Successful use of acitretin in conjunction with narrowband ultraviolet B phototherapy in a child with severe pustular psoriasis, von Zumbusch type. Br J Dermatol 2004;151(4):912–6.
71. Tan SY, Buzney E, Mostaghimi A. Trends in phototherapy utilization among Medicare beneficiaries in the United States, 2000 to 2015. J Am Acad Dermatol 2018;79(4):672–9.
72. Brecher AR, Orlow SJ. Oral retinoid therapy for dermatologic conditions in children and adolescents. J Am Acad Dermatol 2003;49(2):171–82. quiz 183-176.
73. Roenigk HH Jr, Callen JP, Guzzo CA, et al. Effects of acitretin on the liver. J Am Acad Dermatol 1999;41(4):584–8.
74. An J, Zhang D, Wu J, et al. The acitretin and methotrexate combination therapy for psoriasis vulgaris achieves higher effectiveness and less liver fibrosis. Pharmacol Res 2017;121:158–68.
75. Warren RB, Chalmers RJ, Griffiths CE, et al. Methotrexate for psoriasis in the era of biological therapy. Clin Exp Dermatol 2008;33(5):551–4.
76. Hsu L, Armstrong AW. Anti-drug antibodies in psoriasis: a critical evaluation of clinical significance and impact on treatment response. Expert Rev Clin Immunol 2013;9(10):949–58.
77. van Geel MJ, Oostveen AM, Hoppenreijs EP, et al. Methotrexate in pediatric plaque-type psoriasis: Long-term daily clinical practice results from the Child-CAPTURE registry. J Dermatolog Treat 2015;26(5):406–12.
78. Kaur I, Dogra S, De D, et al. Systemic methotrexate treatment in childhood psoriasis: further experience in 24 children from India. Pediatr Dermatol 2008;25(2):184–8.
79. Al-Hammadi A, Ruszczak Z, Magarinos G, et al. Intermittent use of biologic agents for the treatment of psoriasis in adults. J Eur Acad Dermatol Venereol 2021;35(2):360–7.
80. Paller AS, Siegfried EC, Eichenfield LF, et al. Long-term etanercept in pediatric patients with plaque psoriasis. J Am Acad Dermatol 2010;63(5):762–8.
81. Paller AS, Siegfried EC, Langley RG, et al. Etanercept treatment for children and adolescents with plaque psoriasis. N Engl J Med 2008;358(3):241–51.
82. Paller AS, Siegfried EC, Pariser DM, et al. Long-term safety and efficacy of etanercept in children and adolescents with plaque psoriasis. J Am Acad Dermatol 2016;74(2):280–7. e281-283.
83. Adalimumab [package insert] AbbVie, North Chicago, IL 2016.
84. Subedi S, Gong Y, Chen Y, et al. Infliximab and biosimilar infliximab in psoriasis: efficacy, loss of efficacy, and adverse events. Drug Des Devel Ther 2019;13:2491–502.
85. Landells I, Marano C, Hsu MC, et al. Ustekinumab in adolescent patients age 12 to 17 years with moderate-to-severe plaque psoriasis: results of the randomized phase 3 CADMUS study. J Am Acad Dermatol 2015;73(4):594–603.
86. Philipp S, Menter A, Nikkels AF, et al. Ustekinumab for the treatment of moderate-to-severe plaque psoriasis in paediatric patients (>/= 6 to < 12 years of age): efficacy, safety, pharmacokinetic and biomarker results from the open-label CADMUS Jr study. Br J Dermatol 2020;183(4):664–72.
87. Paller AS, Seyger MMB, Alejandro Magarinos G, et al. Efficacy and safety of ixekizumab in a phase III, randomized, double-blind, placebo-controlled study in paediatric patients with moderate-to-severe plaque psoriasis (IXORA-PEDS). Br J Dermatol 2020;183(2):231–41.
88. Bodemer C, Kaszuba A, Kingo K, et al. Secukinumab demonstrates high efficacy and a favourable safety profile in paediatric patients with severe chronic plaque psoriasis: 52-week results from a Phase 3 double-blind randomized, controlled trial. J Eur Acad Dermatol Venereol 2021;35(4):938–47.

Hormonal Treatment of Acne and Hidradenitis Suppurativa in Adolescent Patients

Ryan M. Svoboda, MD, MS[a], Nanjiba Nawaz, BA[b],
Andrea L. Zaenglein, MD[a,c,*]

KEYWORDS

• Acne • Combined oral contraceptive • Spironolactone • Hormonal therapy • Antiandrogen

KEY POINTS

- Combined oral contraceptives (COCs) are effective in the treatment of adolescent acne in female patients.
- Safe use of COCs requires careful review of medical history for contraindications.
- Consider delaying initiation of COC therapy until 2 years after menarche (or age 14 years) in order to ensure adequate bone acquisition unless clinically indicated.
- Spironolactone is an emerging option for the treatment of adolescent female acne, although data from large, well-controlled trials supporting its efficacy are lacking.
- There is a paucity of data supporting the use of COCs and spironolactone in the treatment of hidradenitis suppurativa, but these agents may be considered adjunctively in combination with other therapies.

INTRODUCTION/HISTORY/DEFINITIONS/BACKGROUND

Hormonal influences play a profound role in maintaining homeostasis of the cutaneous microenvironment, particularly in terms of pilosebaceous unit function.[1,2] In addition to being responsive to hormonal signals released by other organs, such as the adrenal glands and gonads, the pilosebaceous unit has been demonstrated to synthesize androgens both de novo and through metabolism of precursor circulating dehydroepiandrosterone sulfate.[1,3] These cutaneous androgens then play a role in the regulation of sebaceous gland activity by means of an intracrine mechanism.[4]

Beyond being vital to normal cutaneous homeostasis, hormones, particularly androgens, also play a role in the pathogenesis of multiple disorders affecting the pilosebaceous unit, the prototype being acne vulgaris.[5] This is mediated through both increased production of sebum and upregulation of inflammatory cytokines in the local follicular microenvironment.[6] An understanding of the role that androgens play in the pathogenesis of follicular disorders can be leveraged by clinicians treating these conditions. Specifically, hormonal therapy in the form of combined oral contraceptive (COC) pills and the aldosterone receptor antagonist, spironolactone, serves as important therapeutic options for the properly selected patient. This article provides a framework for the use of hormonal therapy for the treatment of dermatologic conditions in the adolescent patient

[a] Penn State/ Hershey Medical Center, Department of Dermatology, 500 University Drive, Hershey, PA 17033, USA; [b] Penn State College of Medicine, 500 University Drive, Hershey, PA 17033, USA; [c] Penn State/ Hershey Medical Center, Departments of Dermatology and Pediatrics, 500 University Drive, Hershey, PA 17033, USA
* Corresponding author. Penn State Milton S. Hershey Medical Center, Department of Dermatology, 500 University Drive, Hershey, PA 17033.
E-mail address: azaenglein@pennstatehealth.psu.edu

Dermatol Clin 40 (2022) 167–178
https://doi.org/10.1016/j.det.2021.12.004
0733-8635/22/© 2021 Elsevier Inc. All rights reserved.

and details important considerations in this specific population.

DISCUSSION

Combined Oral Contraceptive Pills

Mechanism of action

COC are composed of ethinyl estradiol and a variable progestin component. The utility of COC pills in the treatment of acne is achieved through several distinct, but complementary, mechanisms, largely related to the action of the estrogen component. First, COCs exert a negative feedback signal on the hypothalamic-pituitary-gonadal axis, suppressing the production of luteinizing hormone, thereby decreasing endogenous androgen synthesis.[7] Although total serum testosterone is reduced via this mechanism, bioavailable (ie, free) testosterone, which represents the clinically important fraction of total testosterone free to exert its effects on the pilosebaceous unit via binding to the androgen receptor, is further lowered in the setting of COC treatment because of an approximately 4-fold upregulation of sex hormone binding globulin.[8] These mechanisms together lead to an approximately 60% reduction in the levels of circulating free testosterone.[7] Decreased follicular concentrations of free testosterone result in diminished binding to and activation of sebaceous gland androgen receptors, thus reducing sebum production.

The effect of the progestin component of COCs on acne is less well understood. In terms of their function as an active ingredient of COCs, progestins serve to provide a more consistent antiovulatory effect and also prevent adverse effects related to long-term exposure to unopposed estrogen (eg, development of endometrial cancer).[9,10] However, certain progestins also have intrinsic androgenic activity through their ability to cross-react with the androgen receptor and thus could theoretically worsen disorders of the folliculosebaceous unit, such as acne.[11] First generation (estranes), second generation (gonanes), and third generation all are derived from testosterone and thus do have some level of inherent androgenic activity, which could theoretically lead to worsening of acne, although when combined with estrogen derivatives, this has not been a particularly practical concern.[12,13] However, progestin-only methods of contraception have been shown to have a negative effect on acne in some patients.[14] Data do suggest that third-generation progestins have decreased androgenic properties compared with first- and second-generation compounds.[15,16] The novel fourth-generation progestin, drospirenone, is a derivative of spironolactone that demonstrates both antimineralocorticoid and antiandrogenic properties[17]. The results of a comparative in vitro dose-response analysis found that drospirenone and other fourth-generation progestins, nestorone and nomegestrol acetate, have a net antiandrogenic effect and are more similar to natural progesterone than earlier-generation progestins.[18] Currently, 4 COCs are specifically approved by the Food and Drug Administration (FDA) for the treatment of acne. **Table 1** lists select common contraceptives and their components.

Efficacy in acne

Multiple randomized controlled trials (RCTs) have assessed the efficacy of COCs in the treatment of acne. A meta-analysis of 31 trials, accounting for 12,579 patients, found that 9 out of 10 RCTs comparing the efficacy of COCs to a placebo demonstrated a statistically significant improvement in acne in patients treated with COCs.[19] Progestins examined were levonorgestrel, norethindrone acetate, norgestimate, drospirenone, dienogest, and chlormadinone acetate (the latter 2 are not currently available in the United States). Outcomes improved in COC-treated patients included lesion counts (total, inflammatory, and noninflammatory), physician-assessed severity (eg, Investigator Global Assessment), and patient-reported outcomes. Several studies combined in this meta-analysis also directly compared the efficacy of different COC formulations differing in terms of the progestin component. Because of the heterogeneity of the studies and the smaller sample sizes for comparison of the different formulations, definitive conclusions were difficult to draw in terms of comparative effectiveness of different COCs.[19] Despite this, one included study comparing 2 formulations approved by the FDA for the treatment of acne did suggest that the combination of drospirenone/ethinyl estradiol may be more effective than norgestimate/ethinyl estradiol.[20] However, it is difficult to make generalized recommendations for specific formulations in terms of efficacy alone, because of the lack of high-quality comparative data.

A more recent meta-analysis aimed to compare the efficacy of COCs with oral antibiotics in the treatment of acne, given the common use of the latter and the controversies surrounding antibiotic stewardship. This combined study of 32 RCTs found that both COCs and oral antibiotics offered statistically significant reduction in total, inflammatory, and noninflammatory lesion counts compared with placebo after 3 and 6 months of treatment.[21] Patients treated with oral antibiotics

Table 1
Select combined oral contraceptives[68]

Estrogen/Dose(mg)	Progestin/Dose (mg)	Additional Component	Brand[a]	Progestin Generation
Monophasic				
EE/0.02	Drospirenone/3	-	Yaz[b] Yasmin	Fourth
EE/0.03	Desogestrel/0.15		Apri	Second
EE/0.02	Drospirenone/3	Levomefolate, Calcium	Beyaz[b]	Fourth
EE/0.035	Norgestimate/0.25	-	Ortho-Cyclen	Third
EE/0.01	Norethindrone acetate/1	Ferrous fumarate	Lo Loestrin Fe	First
EE/0.02	Norethindrone acetate/1	Ferrous fumarate	Junel FE	First
EE/0.025	Norethindrone acetate/0.8	Ferrous fumarate	Generess FE	First
EE/0.02 0.035 0.03	Norethindrone acetate/1 0.5 1.5	-	Junel 21	First
EE/0.035	Norethindrone acetate/0.5	-	Necon 0.5	First
EE/0.03	Norethindrone acetate/1.5	-	Microgestin 1.5	First
EE/0.02 0.03	Levonorgestrel/0.1 0.15	-	Lessina Aviane Lutera Portia	Second
EE/0.03	Norgestrel/0.3		Low-Ogestrel	Third
EE/0.035	Norgestimate/0.25		Sprintec	Third
Biphasic				
EE/0.035	Norethindrone/0.5/1	-	Necon 10/11	First
EE/0.02/0.01	Desogestrel/0.15/0	-	Kariva	Second
Triphasic				
EE/0.035	Norgestimate/0.18/0.215/0.25	-	Ortho Tri-Cyclen[b] Trinessa	Third
EE/0.025	Norgestimate/0.18/0.215/0.25		Ortho Tri-Cyclen Lo	Third
EE/0.025	Desogestrel/0.1/0.125/0.15	-	Cyclessa	Second
EE/0.035	Norethindrone/0.5/0.75/1	-	Necon 7/7/7	First
EE/0.02/0.03/0.035	Norethindrone 1		Estrostep	First
EE/0.03/0.04/0.03	Levonorgestrel/0.05/0.075/0.125	-	Enpresse	Second
Extended Cycle				
EE/0.03	Levonorgestrel/0.15	-	Jolessa Seasonale	Second
EE/0.03/0.01	Levonorgestrel/0.15/0	-	Seasonique	Second
EE/0.02/0.01	Levonorgestrel/0.1/0	-	LoSeasonique	Second

Abbreviation: EE, ethinyl estradiol.
[a] Numerous generics and brands available; commonly used versions listed.
[b] FDA approved for use in acne vulgaris.

did demonstrate slightly greater reduction in mean inflammatory lesion count at 3 months compared with those treated with COCs (53.2% vs 35.6% reduction), but this comparative benefit was lost by 6 months.[21] Because of the concerns with prolonged antibiotic use for the treatment of acne (eg, development of antibiotic resistance), the investigators therefore concluded that COCs may be a more appropriate first-line treatment in properly selected female patients who may require long-term therapy.

Efficacy in hidradenitis suppurativa

Hormonal influences also likely play a role in the pathogenesis of hidradenitis suppurativa (HS), as evidenced by variations in disease severity with the menstrual cycle, with up to 44% to 57% of female patients reporting flares during the premenstrual period.[22,23] Similarly, the observations that pregnancy can lead to both remittance and exacerbation of HS activity, and that menopause leads to resolution of symptoms in up to 48% of women, support the notion that sex hormones play a role in the complex pathophysiologic mechanisms underpinning this disease.[24] Despite these observations, however, the evidence supporting the use of COCs in adolescents with HS is mostly anecdotal and has largely been extrapolated from the acne literature.[25] The North American clinical management guidelines for HS, although acknowledging the lack of quality data in this arena, recommend consideration of estrogen-containing combination oral contraceptives in appropriately selected female patients with HS.[26] Based mostly on existing anecdotal data, this expert consensus recommends avoiding contraceptive agents containing progesterone-only because of the potential to worsen the symptoms of HS.

Safety in adolescents—myths and controversies

Several potential adverse effects must be taken into account when considering the use of COCs for the treatment of dermatologic conditions, specifically in the pediatric population. In addition, patients and their parents will occasionally have concerns with initiating treatment, and it is important to elicit these underlying apprehensions and dispel any myths (**Table 2**).

One of the most common misconceptions regarding the use of COCs is that they lead to weight gain. Prior survey studies have found that up to 75% of women believe weight gain to be a side effect of COC use.[27] More concerning, in one study, 68% of respondents reported being counseled by their health care provider on the possibility of weight gain.[28] Despite this common belief of both patients and providers, there is currently a lack of evidence documenting a clear association between COC use and weight gain. In fact, a Cochrane review including 49 trials did not find any evidence to support a major effect on weight in women taking COCs.[29] Because of the fact that only 4 of the included studies involved

Table 2
Combined oral contraceptive pills—myths and controversies

Myth/Controversy	Current Data
"If I start an oral contraceptive pill, I will experience significant weight gain."	• No evidence to support risk of large weight gain in women started on COC therapy[29] • Insufficient data to definitively exclude the possibility of a small change in weight with COC use[29]
"I can't take my doxycycline since I'm on the pill because there is an interaction."	• Rifamycin antibiotics (including rifampin) may reduce the efficacy of COCs because of increased hepatic metabolism of the latter[30] • Nonrifamycin antibiotics (including doxycycline) have not been demonstrated to have an effect on the efficacy or toxicity of COCs[31]
"Oral contraceptives cause cancer."	• COC use has been associated with decreased risk of endometrial and ovarian cancer, with benefits persisting up to 35 y after discontinuation[33,34] • There is a slight increase in incidence of breast and cervical cancer in active COC users, but this risk normalizes 2–5 y after stopping therapy[33,34]
"I smoke cigarettes so I cannot take an oral contraceptive."	• Smoking is an absolute contraindication for COC in patients older than 35 y ($\geq$15 cigarettes per day), but is a precaution in younger patients[69]

the use of either a placebo group or a control group not using contraception, there was insufficient evidence for the investigators to conclude that there is no possibility of a small change in weight with COC use.[29] However, patients should be counseled that there is no strong evidence to support an association with weight gain, and that there more clearly is no significant risk of a large change in weight attributed to the use of COCs. Proper counseling in this regard is imperative to ensure that patient concerns are addressed, in an effort to maximize adherence to the therapeutic regimen.

Another common misunderstanding surrounding the use of COCs is the potential interaction with antibiotics. This is particularly pertinent to consider in patients using hormonal therapy for the treatment of dermatologic conditions, such as acne or HS, as antibiotics often play in important role in the management of these conditions. Although it is commonly thought that antibiotics can reduce the efficacy of hormone-based contraceptives, only rifamycin antibiotics (eg, rifampin and rifabutin), potent inducers of hepatic cytochrome P450 enzymes, have been shown to alter pharmacokinetic outcomes and reduce systemic exposure to the active hormones.[30] Specifically, a systematic review of 29 studies aimed at determining the pharmacokinetic impact of non-rifamycin antibiotics on hormonal contraception did not find any evidence of either decreased efficacy or increased toxicity of either therapy.[31,32] Importantly, two of the studies considered in this review assessed the possible effects of doxycycline in patients on contraception and found none.[31] Because of the clinical significance and importance of these data, the American College of Obstetrics and Gynecology includes these data in their practice bulletin on the use of hormonal contraception in women with coexisting medical conditions.[32]

Because of the hormonal influences on certain cancers of the female reproductive organs, it is not uncommon for adolescent patients or their parents to raise concerns over the potential for an increase in long-term risk of malignancy. However, the existing evidence does not support a link between COC use and an increased long-term risk of cancer. Specifically, the UK Royal College of General Practitioners' Oral Contraception Study, which followed 46,022 women subjects for up to 44 years, found a decrease in the incidence of endometrial (incidence rate ratio 0.66, 99% confidence interval [CI], 0.48–0.89) and ovarian (incidence rate ratio, 0.67; 99% CI, 0.50–0.89) cancer in ever-users compared with never-users of COCs.[33] Although there was a slightly higher incidence of breast and cervical cancers in current and recent users of COCs compared with never-users and those with a remote history of use, the increased risk dissipated after 5 years of discontinuation.[33] A larger study of 256,661 women found similar results, although in this study the slight increase in the odds of developing breast cancer in women treated with COCs (odds ratio, 1.10; 95% CI, 1.03–1.17) was only noted to persist to 2 years out from discontinuation of therapy. Furthermore, the benefit of reduction in endometrial and ovarian cancers was noted to remain statistically significant out to 35 years.[34] Because breast cancer and cervical cancer are not particularly common in the adolescent age group and the slight increase in risk appears to resolve over time, patients can be counseled that use of COCs for the treatment of adolescent acne carries very little tangible risk of malignancy.

Safety in adolescents—considerations

Despite the overall well-tolerated nature of COCs, adverse events do occur, and particular considerations must be taken into account when prescribing these agents for the treatment of dermatologic conditions in adolescents. Common side effects of COCs include headache, nausea, and breast tenderness, although these often resolve with continued use. Intermenstrual bleeding is another commonly reported phenomenon and may possibly be decreased with the use of third-generation progestin-containing formulations, commonly used for acne and HS.[35]

Estrogen is a primary regulator of bone metabolism, and adequate levels of estradiol are required to ensure adequate bone density development during adolescence; if levels are too low, bone resorption results. Although COCs supply exogenous estrogen, mean circulating levels of endogenous estradiol are lower, as the COC prevents the normal midcycle spike in estrogen needed for ovulation. Bone mass acquisition during adolescence is an important predictor of overall bone health as an adult.[36] Therefore, concern has been raised regarding whether the relatively low doses of estrogen in most COC formulations provide for sufficient bone mass acquisition in adolescents.[37] A systematic review sponsored by the National Osteoporosis Foundation found 8 observational studies and no RCT assessing the impact of COCs on bone health in adolescents.[38] Of these, one study of 122 adolescent women revealed that women who were maintained on COCs for more than 2 years demonstrated a trend toward lesser increase in bone mineral density of the lumbar spine compared with those not treated with COCs and those treated for less than 2 years.[39] Another study of 41 COC users and 26 control subjects found that control subjects experienced a significantly greater increase in both bone mineral content and bone mineral density of the lumbar spine over the course of a year.[40] However, the other 6 studies did not reveal a significant difference in bone mass acquisition between COC-treated patients and controls. Overall, the investigators of the National Osteoporosis Foundation study concluded that there is only a low level of evidence (grade D) supporting a negative effect of oral contraceptives on the bone health of adolescent women.[38] An expert consensus statement published in the official journal of the American Academy of Pediatrics does state that owing to concerns regarding bone mass acquisition, consideration can be given to withholding COC use in adolescents until 1 year after the onset of menses (grade C recommendation).[37] Similarly, the American Academy of Dermatology clinical practice guidelines for the treatment of acne recommend avoiding COC use within 2 years of menarche or in patients under the age of 14 years, unless there is a strong clinical indication to start therapy.[12] Additional considerations that may influence the decision to initiate COC therapy include if the patient has heavy or painful menses.

In addition to these overall recommendations, there has been concern regarding the impact of the precise formulation of COCs on bone mass. As bone mass is negatively impacted by lower levels of serum estradiol, low estrogen COC formulations (containing <30 μg ethinyl estradiol), which are associated with lower mean serum estradiol levels than higher estrogen formulations (≥ 30 μg ethinyl estradiol), may be more detrimental in this regard.[41] Accordingly, data from a large multicenter RCT of more than 1300 adolescents reveal decreased lumbosacral bone mass deposition in subjects randomized to contraception containing 20 μg of ethinyl estradiol compared with those taking a formulation with 30 μg of ethinyl estradiol.[42] Therefore, in terms of reducing risk of future osteopenia, COCs containing 30 μg or more of ethinyl estradiol are preferred.[36]

Venous thromboembolism (VTE) is a potential serious adverse effect of COC treatment and in the past has largely been attributed to the estrogen component of therapy. Indeed, the relative risk of VTE is increased with higher dosages of ethinyl estradiol contained within a COC.[43] For this reason, the concentrations of ethinyl estradiol in commercially available COCs have decreased over time. The contribution of the progestin component of COCs to the risk of VTE has been more hotly debated, although there are data to suggest that formulations containing a third-generation progestin (eg, norgestimate) do portend a slightly higher risk compared with those that include a first- or second-generation agent.[43,44] Furthermore, the second-generation progestin, levonorgestrel, specifically, appears to have the lowest risk of VTE, according to a Cochrane review of 25 publications, although it should be noted that the combination of ethinyl estradiol and levonorgestrel is not currently FDA approved for the treatment of acne in the United States.[45] The results of a more recent meta-analysis suggest that the risk of VTE with fourth-generation (eg, drospirenone) progestin-containing COCs is similar to that of formulations including third-generation progestins, but again, the overall risk was noted to vary only slightly based on progestin class.[46]

The effect of COC use on the risk of arterial thrombosis is less well defined compared with the risk of VTE. The baseline risk of cardiovascular and cerebrovascular insult is relatively low in the adolescent population, and therefore, COC use likely does not lead to a substantial risk of arterial thrombosis in healthy individuals within this group.[47,48] However, a Cochrane review did reveal an overall increase in the risk of myocardial infarction and ischemic stroke in COC users aged 18 to 50 years versus nonusers (Relative Risk, 1.6 and 1.7, respectively).[49] As with the risk of VTE, the incidence of arterial thrombosis does appear directly proportional to the dose of estrogen contained within the COC. However, in contradistinction to the risk of VTE, the incidence of arterial thrombosis does not appear to vary with progestin type.[49] As cigarette smoking, hypertension, and migraine with aura increase the risk of ischemic stroke, COC use for the treatment of acne should be avoided in adolescents with these risk factors.[47] In addition to the risk of ischemic stroke, COC use has also demonstrated an association with a slightly increased risk of hemorrhagic stroke secondary to subarachnoid hemorrhage. This risk is increased in patients taking COCs containing higher concentrations of estrogen and in those with certain comorbidities (ie, current smoking status, hypertension, migraine with aura).[50] Overall, the risk is very low in the adolescent population but must be considered in patients with these coexisting risk factors.

Recommendations

COCs are a valuable option for the treatment of acne in adolescent women and are recommended in the American Academy of Dermatology clinical practice guidelines as an adjunctive treatment consideration for moderate to severe acne (strength of recommendation = A; **Table 3**).[12]

Table 3
Published recommendations for the use of hormonal therapies in the treatment of acne and hidradenitis suppurativa[12,26]

	Acne[a]		Hidradenitis Suppurativa[b]	
Agent	Strength of Recommendation	Level of Evidence	Strength of Recommendation	Level of Evidence
Combined oral contraceptives	A	I	C	II
Spironolactone	B	II	C	III

[a] 2016 American Academy of Dermatology Clinical Practice Guidelines.
[b] 2019 US and Canadian Hidradenitis Suppurativa Foundation Joint Guidelines.

These agents may also be useful in select patients with HS as adjunctive therapy (see **Table 3**). Before initiation, baseline blood pressure should be measured. According to World Health Organization guidelines, COC use is contraindicated in patients with baseline blood pressure ≥160/100 mm Hg and should be initiated cautiously in those with a milder degree of hypertension (140–159/90–99 mm Hg). Other situations in which COC use is not recommended, that may pertain to adolescents, include diabetes with end-organ damage, history of VTE, recent major surgery with prolonged immobilization, history of migraine with focal neurologic deficit (ie, aura), and active viral hepatitis (**Box 1**).[13] It is important to counsel patients that although COCs can be started at any point throughout the menstrual cycle, protection from pregnancy will not be established until after 7 days unless initiated within 5 days of the first day of menses. It is also vital to educate patients that in terms of efficacy, it typically takes approximately 3 months for significant improvement in acne to be seen (and perhaps longer for HS).

Beyond being used for the direct treatment of cutaneous disease, COCs can play an adjunctive role in management as a method of preventing pregnancy in instances where the primary treatment is known to be teratogenic. For example, COCs are often used in adolescent female acne patients being treated with isotretinoin, as the iPledge program requires that all sexually active patients of childbearing potential use 2 forms of birth control. Although it has not been specifically studied, it is mechanistically possible that the addition of a COC to isotretinoin therapy may lead to quicker resolution of acne. It is important to know that estradiol and isotretinoin are both metabolized largely via hepatic cytochrome P450 3A4, and that isotretinoin does lead to a slight potential decrease in plasma concentrations of ethinyl estradiol.[51] Despite this, pharmacodynamic changes have not been noted, but this piece of pharmacokinetic data does suggest the importance of the second method of contraception in patients taking isotretinoin who are heterosexually active.[51]

Box 1
World Health Organization contraindications to combined oral contraceptive therapy

Absolute contraindications
- Current pregnancy
- Current breastfeeding if less than 6 weeks postpartum
- Current breast cancer
- Current smoker (≥15 cigarettes per day) *and* age ≥35 years[a]
- Diabetes greater than 20 years' duration or with end-organ damage
- History of venous thromboembolism
- Hypertension
  - Systolic blood pressure ≥160 mm Hg
  - Diastolic blood pressure ≥100 mm Hg
- Ischemic coronary disease
- Valvular heart disease with complications
- History of stroke
- Migraine with aura (focal neurologic deficit)
- Active viral hepatitis
- Decompensated cirrhosis

Relative contraindications
- Current symptomatic gall bladder disease
- Anticonvulsant therapy
- Migraine without aura *and* age ≥35 years[a]

[a] Not a consideration in adolescent populations.

Similarly, COCs may be helpful as a method of pregnancy prevention in adolescent patients with inflammatory dermatoses who are being treated with other known teratogens, such as methotrexate or mycophenolate mofetil. In cases such as these, the expected benefit of COC use would be solely in terms of birth control.

Spironolactone

Mechanism of action

Spironolactone is a potent mineralocorticoid receptor antagonist that was initially developed as a potassium-sparing diuretic and has played a larger role in the treatment of progressive heart failure and refractory hypertension.[52] In addition to its antimineralocorticoid activity, spironolactone also exhibits antiandrogen effects, through both competitive antagonistic binding to the androgen receptor and decreased testosterone production.[53,54] Furthermore, spironolactone may secondarily inhibit cutaneous 5α-reductase, thus leading to decreased conversion of testosterone to the more potent dihydrotestosterone.[55] Because of these antiandrogenic effects, the use of spironolactone in an "off-label" manner has become commonplace in the treatment of disorders centered on pathology of the pilosebaceous unit.

Efficacy in acne

Several studies have investigated the therapeutic benefit of spironolactone in the treatment of acne. A recent single-center cohort study of 80 adolescent women treated with spironolactone (median dose, 100 mg daily) demonstrated a greater than 50% improvement in acne in 58.8% of subjects, with 22.5% experiencing a complete response.[56] Similarly, a retrospective series of 403 women from a single center revealed a reduction in Comprehensive Acne Severity Scale score in 75.5% of subjects with facial acne treated with spironolactone, although this latter study included only adult women (median age, 26 years).[57] This study did demonstrate similar efficacy of spironolactone in the treatment of truncal acne as well.[57] Despite this, data from large RCT are relatively lacking. A small randomized, double-blind, placebo-controlled crossover study of 21 women did demonstrate a statistically significant improvement in subjective assessment of acne and inflammatory lesion count during treatment with spironolactone.[58] Overall, data supporting the use of spironolactone in the treatment of female acne are promising but not sufficient to draw definitive conclusions, and more studies are needed in this area, particularly in the adolescent population. Despite this, a working group convened by the American Academy of Dermatology, taking into consideration the existing data as well as personal experience and expert opinion, recommends the use of spironolactone in the treatment of acne in select female patients (see **Table 3**).[12]

Efficacy in hidradenitis suppurativa

There are little primary data examining the efficacy of spironolactone in treating this condition. A retrospective study of 20 female patients (including 5 adolescents) demonstrated a reduction in Physician's Global Assessment in 85% of subjects after 3 months of treatment. Of these, 11/20 (55%) achieved complete remission of disease activity. Patients with mild disease were more likely to achieve complete clearance.[59] Overall, the lack of quality data in this arena represents a knowledge gap, and although spironolactone likely represents a low-risk option for women with HS, its use currently receives only a "grade C" recommendation from the North American clinical management guideline working group (see **Table 3**).[26]

Safety in adolescents

Spironolactone has demonstrated an excellent safety record in the long-term treatment of acne. A study of 91 women maintained on spironolactone for a mean of 28.5 months demonstrated no serious adverse effects related to spironolactone over an 8-year follow-up period.[60] This same study did reveal that although side effects are common and dose dependent (occurring in 59% of patients), they only resulted in premature discontinuation of treatment 15% of the time.[60] The most common side effects attributed to spironolactone are slight diuresis and menstrual irregularities, occurring in 29% and 22% of patients, respectively. Menstrual adverse effects are decreased by the concomitant use of COCs, and given the efficacy of the latter in the treatment of acne (and to a lesser degree, HS), the use of these medications together can be an effective strategy.[57] Other common side effects of spironolactone include breast tenderness, breast enlargement, fatigue, headache, and lightheadedness.[60] Importantly, no significant long-term safety concerns were reported in this study, and no patients were diagnosed with breast, ovarian, endometrial, or cervical carcinoma. Because of the largely theoretic risk of undervirilization of the male fetus and the theoretic risk of intrauterine growth retardation, spironolactone is considered FDA pregnancy category C and should be discontinued if pregnancy develops.[61]

Because of the potassium-sparing nature of antimineralocorticoid agents, the potential for the development of hyperkalemia has been a persistent concern of both patients and health care providers. However, a large study showed no difference in the rate of hyperkalemia in a group of 974 healthy young adult women ages 18 to 45 years (mean age, 27.5 years) prescribed spironolactone for the treatment of acne compared with 1165 healthy control subjects.[62] In addition, studies have not revealed significant hyperkalemia in patients being concomitantly treated with spironolactone and COCs containing the spironolactone analogue, drospirenone.[63] Therefore, in the absence of underlying renal, adrenal, or hepatic disease, routine serum potassium monitoring is not essential for healthy young adult women prescribed spironolactone for the treatment of acne.[62] This recommendation can be extrapolated to healthy adolescents as well.

THE EFFECTS OF OTHER CONTRACEPTIVES ON ACNE AND HIDRADENITIS SUPPURATIVA

A variety of other modalities that contain a hormonal component are used for the purpose of contraception. Because of the varying degrees of the estrogen and progestin components, these agents have varied effects on dermatologic conditions and have been most well studied in acne vulgaris. Although these agents are not usually chosen solely for the indication of treating dermatologic disease, it is important for the clinician to be aware of the possible impact of these other forms of contraception on acne and HS, as multidisciplinary discussion may be required to determine the optimal form of contraception for a given patient. **Table 4** details the effects of alternative forms of hormonal contraception on acne and HS. Further research is needed, particularly in the realm of HS, to better characterize the effects of these alternative forms of contraception on preexisting skin disease.[14,64,65] It is important to emphasize that in individual patients, progesterone-only contraceptives, such as drospirenone, have been self-reported to improve acne and HS, but in a greater proportion of these patients, the net effect appears to be negative.[14,65] Therefore, it is essential to tailor management on a patient-by-patient basis, depending on the possible benefits of a given contraception modality and the severity of preexisting skin disease.

Table 4
Other contraceptive forms and effects on acne and hidradenitis suppurativa[14]

Type	Hormonal Component	Brand[a]	Effect on Acne[14]	Effect on HS[64,65]
Injectable (progestin only)	Depot medroxyprogesterone	Depot-Provera	–	–
Pill (progestin only)	Drospirenone pill Norethindrone pill	Slynd Camila, Errin, Heather, Micronor	N/A[b] –[c]	N/A[b] –[c]
Transdermal contraceptive patch	Norelgestromin and ethinyl estradiol	Xulane, Evra	+[c]	+/–
Combined hormonal vaginal ring	Etonogestrel and ethinyl estradiol	Annovera NuvaRing	+[c]	+/–
Long-acting reversible contraception	Etonogestrel Levonorgestrel	Nexplanon Norplant	– D/C	+/– D/C
Intrauterine device	Levonorgestrel None (copper)	Mirena, Skyla Paragard	– N/A	– N/A

Abbreviations: –, may worsen condition; +, may improve condition; +/–, equivocal effect; D/C, discontinued; N/A, data not available.

[a] Numerous generics and brands available; commonly used versions listed.

[b] Newly approved formulation; package insert lists acne as an adverse event in 3.8% of individuals.[70]

[c] Existing data are not sufficient to draw definitive conclusions; presumed effect based on limited data/extrapolation from data on other contraceptive formulations with similar hormonal components.

New Therapies

Clascoterone 1% cream is a topical androgen receptor inhibitor approved by the FDA in August 2020 for the treatment of acne vulgaris in patients aged 12 and older.[66] Clascoterone is unique in that it will be the first commercially available topical antiandrogen treatment and can safely be used in male patients without significant concern for systemic antiandrogen side effects. Although long-term safety and efficacy data are not yet available, data from phase III clinical trials demonstrate a statistically significant reduction compared with vehicle in inflammatory and noninflammatory lesions from baseline (−19.3 vs −15.5 and −19.4 vs −13.0 for inflammatory and noninflammatory lesions, respectively), in addition to a favorable safety profile.[67] Despite the fact that this trial included patients ranging from age 10 to 58 years, the sample heavily favored the adolescent population (median age, 18). Although postmarket data will be essential, clascoterone cream may be a promising addition to the clinician's arsenal of hormonal agents for the treatment of acne in adolescents.

SUMMARY

Hormonal therapies are increasingly used for the treatment of acne and HS in the adolescent population. COCs have been extensively studied in adolescents with age-specific concerns regarding long-term osteoporosis risk identified. Data on the efficacy of spironolactone in teens with acne and HS are lacking, with support for its use primarily extrapolated from studies in adult women. The safety and efficacy of both COCs and spironolactone in younger adolescent patients need to be further studied.

CLINICS CARE POINTS

- Estrogen-containing combined oral contraceptives are effective in the treatment of adolescent acne in female patients.
- Combined oral contraceptives with estrogen doses of 30 to 35 μg and third- or fourth-generation progestins are recommended for adolescents with acne and hidradenitis suppurativa. Consider delaying initiation of combined oral contraceptive therapy until 2 years after menarche (or age 14), in order to ensure adequate bone mass acquisition.
- Safe use of combined oral contraceptives requires careful review of medical history for contraindications.
- Combined oral contraceptives should be avoided in patients with a history of venous thromboembolism, complicated valvular heart disease (rare among adolescents), and focal neurologic deficit (including migraine with aura).
- Spironolactone appears to be a safe and well-tolerated option for the treatment of adolescent female acne, although data regarding safe use in younger adolescents are particularly lacking.
- There is a paucity of data supporting the use of combined oral contraceptives and spironolactone in the treatment of hidradenitis suppurativa, but these agents may be considered adjunctively in combination with traditional therapies.

DISCLOSURES

Ryan M. Svoboda, MD and Nanjiba Nawaz, BA have no relevant financial disclosures.

Andrea L. Zaenglein, MD: Abbvie (investigator), Arcutis (investigator), Cassiopea (advisory board), Incyte (investigator), Pfizer (investigator, consultant), Regeneron (advisory board), Verrica (advisory board), *Pediatric Dermatology* (editor-in-chief), UptoDate (author).

REFERENCES

1. Chen W-C, Zouboulis CC. Hormones and the pilosebaceous unit. Dermatoendocrinology 2009;1:81–6.
2. Chen W, Thiboutot D, Zouboulis CC. Cutaneous androgen metabolism: basic research and clinical perspectives. J Invest Dermatol 2002;119:992–1007.
3. Thiboutot D, Jabara S, McAllister JM, et al. Human skin is a steroidogenic tissue: steroidogenic enzymes and cofactors are expressed in epidermis, normal sebocytes, and an immortalized sebocyte cell line (SEB-1). J Invest Dermatol 2003;120:905–14.
4. Labrie F, Luu-The V, Labrie C, et al. Intracrinology and the skin. Horm Res 2000;54:218–29.
5. Ju Q, Tao T, Hu T, et al. Sex hormones and acne. Clin Dermatol 2017;35:130–7.
6. Lee WJ, Jung HD, Chi SG, et al. Effect of dihydrotestosterone on the upregulation of inflammatory cytokines in cultured sebocytes. Arch Dermatol Res 2010;302:429–33.
7. Thorneycroft IH, Stanczyk FZ, Bradshaw KD, et al. Effect of low-dose oral contraceptives on androgenic markers and acne. Contraception 1999;60:255–62.

8. Panzer C, Wise S, Fantini G, et al. Impact of oral contraceptives on sex hormone-binding globulin and androgen levels: a retrospective study in women with sexual dysfunction. J Sex Med 2006;3:104–13.
9. Barros B, Thiboutot D. Hormonal therapies for acne. Clin Dermatol 2017;35:168–72.
10. Apgar BS, Greenberg G. Using progestins in clinical practice. Am Fam Physician 2000;62:1839–46, 1849–50.
11. Jones EE. Androgenic effects of oral contraceptives: implications for patient compliance. Am J Med 1995;98:116s–9s.
12. Zaenglein AL, Pathy AL, Schlosser BJ, et al. Guidelines of care for the management of acne vulgaris. J Am Acad Dermatol 2016;74:945–73.e33.
13. Arrington EA, Patel NS, Gerancher K, et al. Combined oral contraceptives for the treatment of acne: a practical guide. Cutis 2012;90:83–90.
14. David Lortscher M, Shehla Admani M, Nancy Satur M, et al. Hormonal contraceptives and acne: a retrospective analysis of 2147 patients. J Drugs Dermatol 2016;15:670–4.
15. Phillips A, Demarest K, Hahn DW, et al. Progestational and androgenic receptor binding affinities and in vivo activities of norgestimate and other progestins. Contraception 1990;41:399–410.
16. Bosanac SS, Trivedi M, Clark AK, et al. Progestins and acne vulgaris: a review. Dermatol Online J 2018;24.
17. Mathur R, Levin O, Azziz R. Use of ethinylestradiol/drospirenone combination in patients with the polycystic ovary syndrome. Ther Clin Risk Manag 2008;4:487.
18. Louw-du Toit R, Perkins MS, Hapgood JP, et al. Comparing the androgenic and estrogenic properties of progestins used in contraception and hormone therapy. Biochem Biophys Res Commun 2017;491:140–6.
19. Arowojolu AO, Gallo MF, Lopez LM, et al. Combined oral contraceptive pills for treatment of acne. Cochrane Database Syst Rev 2012;(7):Cd004425.
20. Thorneycroft I H, Gollnick H, Schellschmidt I. Superiority of a combined contraceptive containing drospirenone to a triphasic preparation containing norgestimate in acne treatment. Cutis 2004;74:123–30.
21. Koo EB, Petersen TD, Kimball AB. Meta-analysis comparing efficacy of antibiotics versus oral contraceptives in acne vulgaris. J Am Acad Dermatol 2014;71:450–9.
22. von der Werth JM, Williams HC. The natural history of hidradenitis suppurativa. J Eur Acad Dermatol Venereol 2000;14:389–92.
23. Harrison BJ, Read GF, Hughes LE. Endocrine basis for the clinical presentation of hidradenitis suppurativa. Br J Surg 1988;75:972–5.
24. Kromann CB, Deckers IE, Esmann S, et al. Risk factors, clinical course and long-term prognosis in hidradenitis suppurativa: a cross-sectional study. Br J Dermatol 2014;171:819–24.
25. Clark AK, Quinonez RL, Saric S, et al. Hormonal therapies for hidradenitis suppurativa: review. Dermatol Online J 2017;23.
26. Alikhan A, Sayed C, Alavi A, et al. North American Clinical Management Guidelines for hidradenitis suppurativa: a publication from the United States and Canadian Hidradenitis Suppurativa Foundations: part II: topical, intralesional, and systemic medical management. J Am Acad Dermatol 2019;81:91–101.
27. Turner RM. Most British women use reliable contraceptive methods, but many fear health risks from use. Perspect Sex Reprod Health 1994;26:183.
28. Gaudet LM, Kives S, Hahn PM, et al. What women believe about oral contraceptives and the effect of counseling. Contraception 2004;69:31–6.
29. Gallo MF, Lopez LM, Grimes DA, et al. Combination contraceptives: effects on weight. Cochrane Database Syst Rev 2014;(9):Cd003987.
30. Simmons KB, Haddad LB, Nanda K, et al. Drug interactions between rifamycin antibiotics and hormonal contraception: a systematic review. BJOG 2018;125:804–11.
31. Simmons KB, Haddad LB, Nanda K, et al. Drug interactions between non-rifamycin antibiotics and hormonal contraception: a systematic review. Am J Obstet Gynecol 2018;218:88–97.e14.
32. ACOG Practice Bulletin No. 206: use of hormonal contraception in women with coexisting medical conditions. Obstet Gynecol 2019;133:e128–50.
33. Iversen L, Sivasubramaniam S, Lee AJ, et al. Lifetime cancer risk and combined oral contraceptives: the Royal College of General Practitioners' Oral Contraception Study. Am J Obstet Gynecol 2017;216:580.e1–9.
34. Karlsson T, Johansson T, Höglund J, et al. Time-dependent effects of oral contraceptive use on breast, ovarian and endometrial cancers. Cancer Res 2020.
35. Lawrie TA, Helmerhorst FM, Maitra NK, et al. Types of progestogens in combined oral contraception: effectiveness and side-effects. Cochrane Database Syst Rev 2011;(5):Cd004861.
36. Golden NH. Bones and birth control in adolescent girls. J Pediatr Adolesc Gynecol 2020;33:249–54.
37. Eichenfield LF, Krakowski AC, Piggott C, et al. Evidence-based recommendations for the diagnosis and treatment of pediatric acne. Pediatrics 2013;131(Suppl 3):S163–86.
38. Weaver CM, Gordon CM, Janz KF, et al. The National Osteoporosis Foundation's position statement on peak bone mass development and lifestyle factors: a systematic review and implementation recommendations. Osteoporos Int 2016;27:1281–386.

39. Pikkarainen E, Lehtonen-Veromaa M, Möttönen T, et al. Estrogen-progestin contraceptive use during adolescence prevents bone mass acquisition: a 4-year follow-up study. Contraception 2008;78:226–31.
40. Biason TP, Goldberg TB, Kurokawa CS, et al. Low-dose combined oral contraceptive use is associated with lower bone mineral content variation in adolescents over a 1-year period. BMC Endocr Disord 2015;15:15.
41. Ziglar S, Hunter TS. The effect of hormonal oral contraception on acquisition of peak bone mineral density of adolescents and young women. J Pharm Pract 2012;25:331–40.
42. Gersten J, Hsieh J, Weiss H, et al. Effect of extended 30 μg ethinyl estradiol with continuous low-dose ethinyl estradiol and cyclic 20 μg ethinyl estradiol oral contraception on adolescent bone density: a randomized trial. J Pediatr Adolesc Gynecol 2016;29:635–42.
43. Stegeman BH, de Bastos M, Rosendaal FR, et al. Different combined oral contraceptives and the risk of venous thrombosis: systematic review and network meta-analysis. BMJ 2013;347:f5298.
44. Venous thromboembolic disease and combined oral contraceptives: results of international multicentre case-control study. World Health Organization Collaborative Study of Cardiovascular Disease and Steroid Hormone Contraception. Lancet 1995;346:1575–82.
45. de Bastos M, Stegeman BH, Rosendaal FR, et al. Combined oral contraceptives: venous thrombosis. Cochrane Database Syst Rev 2014;(3):CD010813.
46. Bateson D, Butcher BE, Donovan C, et al. Risk of venous thromboembolism in women taking the combined oral contraceptive: a systematic review and meta-analysis. Aust Fam Physician 2016;45:59–64.
47. Harper JC. Use of oral contraceptives for management of acne vulgaris: practical considerations in real world practice. Dermatol Clin 2016;34:159–65.
48. Organization WH. Cardiovascular disease and steroid contraception: report of a WHO Scientific Group. World Health Organization; 1998. p. 1–89.
49. Roach REJ, Helmerhorst FM, Lijfering WM, et al. Combined oral contraceptives: the risk of myocardial infarction and ischemic stroke. Cochrane Database Syst Rev 2015;2015:CD011054.
50. Xu Z, Yue Y, Bai J, et al. Association between oral contraceptives and risk of hemorrhagic stroke: a meta-analysis of observational studies. Arch Gynecol Obstet 2018;297:1181–91.
51. Hendrix CW, Jackson KA, Jackson KA, et al. The effect of isotretinoin on the pharmacokinetics and pharmacodynamics of ethinyl estradiol and norethindrone. Clin Pharmacol Ther 2004;75:464–75.
52. Lainscak M, Pelliccia F, Rosano G, et al. Safety profile of mineralocorticoid receptor antagonists: spironolactone and eplerenone. Int J Cardiol 2015;200:25–9.
53. Rifka SM, Pita JC, Vigersky RA, et al. Interaction of digitalis and spironolactone with human sex steroid receptors. J Clin Endocrinol Metab 1978;46:338–44.
54. Akamatsu H, Zouboulis CC, Orfanos CE. Spironolactone directly inhibits proliferation of cultured human facial sebocytes and acts antagonistically to testosterone and 5 alpha-dihydrotestosterone in vitro. J Invest Dermatol 1993;100:660–2.
55. Serafini PC, Catalino J, Lobo RA. The effect of spironolactone on genital skin 5 alpha-reductase activity. J Steroid Biochem 1985;23:191–4.
56. Roberts EE, Nowsheen S, Davis DMR, et al. Use of spironolactone to treat acne in adolescent females. Pediatr Dermatol 2021;38:72–6.
57. Garg V, Choi JK, James WD, et al. Long-term use of spironolactone for acne in women: a case series of 403 patients. J Am Acad Dermatol 2021.
58. Muhlemann MF, Carter GD, Cream JJ, et al. Oral spironolactone: an effective treatment for acne vulgaris in women. Br J Dermatol 1986;115:227–32.
59. Lee A, Fischer G. A case series of 20 women with hidradenitis suppurativa treated with spironolactone. Australas J Dermatol 2015;56:192–6.
60. Shaw JC, White LE. Long-term safety of spironolactone in acne: results of an 8-year followup study. J Cutan Med Surg 2002;6:541–5.
61. Riester A, Reincke M. Progress in primary aldosteronism: mineralocorticoid receptor antagonists and management of primary aldosteronism in pregnancy. Eur J Endocrinol 2015;172:R23–30.
62. Plovanich M, Weng QY, Mostaghimi A. Low usefulness of potassium monitoring among healthy young women taking spironolactone for acne. JAMA Dermatol 2015;151:941–4.
63. Krunic A, Ciurea A, Scheman A. Efficacy and tolerance of acne treatment using both spironolactone and a combined contraceptive containing drospirenone. J Am Acad Dermatol 2008;58:60–2.
64. Williams NM, Randolph M, Rajabi-Estarabadi A, et al. Hormonal contraceptives and dermatology. Am J Clin Dermatol 2021;22(1):69–80.
65. Collier EK, Price KN, Grogan TR, et al. Characterizing perimenstrual flares of hidradenitis suppurativa. Int J Womens Dermatol 2020;6:372–6.
66. Kalabalik-Hoganson J, Frey KM, Ozdener-Poyraz AE, et al. Clascoterone: a novel topical androgen receptor inhibitor for the treatment of acne. Ann Pharmacother 2021.
67. Hebert A, Thiboutot D, Stein Gold L, et al. Efficacy and safety of topical clascoterone cream, 1%, for treatment in patients with facial acne: two phase 3 randomized clinical trials. JAMA Dermatol 2020;156:621–30.
68. Contraceptives PO, Role ANP: continuing education for pharmacists & pharmacy technicians.
69. Organization WH, Health WHOR. Medical eligibility criteria for contraceptive use. World Health Organization; 2010.
70. Slynd pacakge insert. Exeltis USA; 2019.

Sweet Syndrome in the Pediatric Population

Danielle McClanahan, MD, Tracy Funk, MD, Alison Small, MD*

KEYWORDS

• Sweet syndrome • Acute febrile neutrophilic dermatosis • Pediatric

KEY POINTS

- Sweet syndrome (SS) diagnostic criteria are based on adult literature and have been extrapolated to pediatric patients.
- Categorizing patients into age groups ranging from birth to less than 3 months (neonatal SS), 3 months to less than 3 years (infantile SS), and 3 years to 18 years (junior SS) is useful for screening for associated diseases of SS.
- Comprehensive long-term management guidelines for pediatric patients with SS are lacking and likely would be of value for providers.

INTRODUCTION

In 1964, Sweet syndrome (SS) was first described by Dr Robert Sweet[1] in a case series of adult female patients presenting with tender cutaneous plaques and nodules and neutrophilic infiltrates on histopathology. Today, the pathophysiology of SS remains unclear but is thought to be due to a hypersensitivity reaction from an underlying inflammatory or infectious state. Pediatric SS typically is diagnosed using criteria created for adult SS patients.[2] Children and adolescents make up 5% to 8% of cases, and there currently are approximately 80 pediatric patients described in the medical literature.[3,4] Significant differences exist between adult and pediatric SS patient populations.[3–7] Given the differences in populations and associated underlying conditions, screening work-up and management recommendations have been proposed for pediatric patients.[3,8] This article summarizes the current medical literature on the topic of pediatric SS and suggests clinical guidelines for evaluation and long-term management of these patients.

BACKGROUND

Categories

SS initially was organized into 5 categories based on underlying etiology, including classic idiopathic, para-inflammatory, paraneoplastic, pregnancy-associated, and drug-related.[5,9] Recently, various investigators have used a simplified categorical system with 3 variants: classic (associated with upper respiratory and gastrointestinal infection, inflammatory bowel disease, or pregnancy), paraneoplastic, and drug related.[4,10,11]

Diagnostic Criteria for Sweet Syndrome

Su and Liu[12] proposed the first diagnostic criteria for SS in 1986 after reviewing available medical literature and applying their criteria to 5 adult cases with an average age of 60 years. In 1994, these criteria were revised by von den Driesch[9] based on a literature review of 38 patients with an average age of 53 years. The investigator made modifications in some of the minor criteria, including required laboratory values, associated conditions, and response to potassium iodide. These often-used diagnostic criteria require both 2 major criteria and 2 minor criteria for diagnosis (**Box 1**).[8,9] These criteria have been extrapolated to pediatric patients despite differences between adult and pediatric populations.

Malignancy-associated Sweet Syndrome

A diagnosis of malignancy-associated SS (MASS) utilizes the diagnostic criteria for SS with the minor

Department of Dermatology, Oregon Health and Science Univeristy, 3303 South Bond Avenue, Center for Health and Healing Building 1, 16th Floor, Portland, OR 97239, USA
* Corresponding author.
E-mail address: smalla@ohsu.edu

Dermatol Clin 40 (2022) 179–190
https://doi.org/10.1016/j.det.2021.12.005
0733-8635/22/© 2021 Elsevier Inc. All rights reserved.

Box 1
Diagnostic criteria for Sweet syndrome

Major criteria[a]

1. Abrupt onset of tender or painful erythematous plaques or nodules occasionally with vesicles, pustules, or bullae
2. Predominantly neutrophilic infiltration in the dermis without leukocytoclastic vasculitis

Minor criteria[a]

1. Preceded by a nonspecific respiratory or gastrointestinal tract infection or vaccination or associated with
   - Inflammatory diseases, such as chronic autoimmune disorders, infections
   - Hemoproliferative disorders or solid malignant tumors
   - Pregnancy
2. Accompanied by periods of general malaise and fever (>38°C)
3. Laboratory values during onset: ESR, greater than 20 mm/h; CRP, positive; segmented-nuclear neutrophils and stabs, greater than 70% in peripheral blood smear; leukocytosis greater than 8000 cells/mm^3 (3 of 4 of these values necessary)
4. Excellent response to treatment with systemic corticosteroids or potassium

[a] Both major and 2 minor criteria are needed for diagnosis.

From von den Driesch P. Sweet's syndrome (acute febrile neutrophilic dermatosis). J Am Acad Dermatol. 1994 Oct;31(4):535-56; quiz 557-60.

criterion of malignancy.[7] Malignancies may be diagnosed prior to and concurrently with SS, although also may be discovered following a diagnosis of SS. Therefore, patients previously thought to have classic SS can be reclassified as MASS, sometimes as late as 11 years later.[7,13] Hospach and colleagues[3] found that pediatric malignancies were diagnosed most often simultaneously with SS but recommended ongoing monitoring in patients with classic SS. Patients with a history of prior malignancy should be evaluated thoroughly, because MASS development can herald recurrence.[14] Some of the paraneoplastic syndromes or malignancies associated with pediatric SS include acute myeloid leukemia, osteosarcoma, Fanconi anemia, aplastic anemia, and myelodysplastic syndrome.[5,15] Although red flags for MASS in adult patients include anemia and thrombocytopenia, these are less helpful in pediatric patients who have been found to have thrombocytosis, in approximately 50% of cases.[5]

Drug-induced Sweet Syndrome

Proposed by Walker and Cohen[16] in 1996, criteria for drug-induced SS (DISS) include abrupt onset of tender erythematous papules or nodules with corresponding histopathologic evidence, fever, or relationship between drug initiation and clinical symptoms; recurrence with rechallenge; and resolution after drug withdrawal or treatment with corticosteroids. The timeline of DISS usually is an exposure 10 days to 14 days before presentation of SS.[17] Distinguishing DISS from MASS or classic SS can be complicated when multiple drugs are used in the treatment of a malignancy, inflammatory bowel disease, infection, or paraneoplastic disorder. A lack of neutrophilia has been documented in many patients with DISS.[16] Overall, DISS is less common in pediatric patients. Some of the drugs that have been implicated in pediatric patients include granulocyte colony-stimulating factor, all-trans-retinoic acid, trimethoprim-sulfamethoxazole, and azathioprine.[5,17,18]

Histiocytoid Sweet Syndrome

Histiocytoid SS (HSS) is an entity that presents similarly to SS, however, histologically is composed of histiocytoid mononuclear cells with myeloperoxidase reactivity rather than mature neutrophils. Thus, it is thought that these cells represent immature myeloid cells, likely neutrophil precursors.[19] There has been controversy regarding whether this variant should be classified as SS because it does not meet the pathologic criteria of typical neutrophilic infiltrates. There is some thought that it may be more strongly related to MASS or DISS in adult patients.[20] Although there are fewer pediatric cases of HSS in the literature, the underlying associations with these cases have not included malignancy. Reported cases have been associated with vaccination[20]; lupus erythematosus[21]; Kawasaki disease; a case of serositis, arthritis, and myocarditis[22]; inflammatory bowel disease[19]; and 1 case of no underlying disease.[23]

INITIAL EVALUATION

Once a diagnosis of SS is considered based on recognition of cutaneous lesions with the classic morphology of SS, initial evaluation includes a thorough physical examination of the skin and mucosa as well as systemic examination (heart, lungs, abdomen, and joints), vital signs, tissue biopsies for histopathologic review and culture to rule out infection, and a laboratory work-up (**Table 1**). Because response to treatment is a criterion in the diagnosis of SS, it should be considered part of the evaluation but is discussed later in the treatment section.

Morphology

Classically, SS skin lesions are erythematous, tender papules, plaques, and nodules that appear abruptly (**Fig. 1**). Pediatric patients may present with atypical lesions. Morphologies described in pediatric SS include vesicles, pustules (**Fig. 2**), bullae (**Fig. 3**), oral ulceration, pseudovesicles, and pathergy (**Fig. 4**).[4,5] Lesions are found most commonly on the limbs (90%), followed by the head and trunk (70% and 25%, respectively).[6]

A rare cutaneous complication of SS is the development of cutis laxa, which may be observed in resolving SS lesions.[24,25] Cutis laxa is more common in children compared with adults, with approximately 30% of pediatric cases developing postinflammatory scarring and/or acquired cutis laxa.[6] Furthermore, 20% of pediatric patients have evidence of pathergy and, of those patients, more than 60% are at risk of postinflammatory scarring or acquired cutis laxa.[6]

Clinical Differential Diagnosis

The clinical differential diagnosis is extensive and includes infection, other neutrophilic dermatoses (bowel bypass–related dermatosis and pyoderma gangrenosum), urticaria, vasculitis, cutaneous lupus, benign or malignant neoplasms, and drug hypersensitivity reactions.[4,7,26] Additionally, pediatric patients who present with bullous SS may mimic other bullous entities, such as bullous impetigo.[24,27]

Histopathology

The classic histopathologic findings in SS are marked papillary dermal edema and neutrophilic infiltration of the dermis without leukocytoclastic vasculitis (LCV).[9] Because the absence of vasculitis on histology is a major required diagnostic criterion, if LCV is present on histopathology, it should be focal and secondary to the primary process without classic findings of primary LCV.[7,14] Occasionally, spongiosis or intraepidermal/subepidermal vesiculation can be observed.[5] The histopathologic differential for SS includes other neutrophilic dermatoses and infection. Immunohistochemical stains and tissue cultures can be helpful in ruling out infection.[14] The histopathologic differential diagnosis also may include panniculitis. Septal and lobular panniculitis have been found in approximately 12% and 5% of cases of known SS, respectively.[28,29]

Associations

It is estimated that 22% to 45% of pediatric SS cases occur following an acute infection; most commonly reported are otitis media and viral upper respiratory or gastrointestinal infection.[3] Chronic inflammatory conditions are associated with approximately 30% to 33% of cases in children and can include inflammatory bowel disease, central nervous system vasculitis, chronic recurrent multifocal osteomyelitis (CRMO), autoimmune hepatitis, metabolic disorders, systemic lupus erythematosus, and subacute lupus erythematosus.[3,5] Approximately 15% to 25% of cases occur in association with a paraneoplastic disease, which are discussed in more detail previously. Finally, 21% to 42% of cases are idiopathic without a known association.[3–7] Common associations can be found in **Table 1**.

Specific associations in neonates with SS include neonatal lupus erythematosus and immunodeficiency.[6,30,31] Additionally, congenital malformations that predispose patients to infection or an inflammatory state can present during this time period. For instance, there have been reports of female neonates with SS between 4 weeks and 6 weeks of age who were found to have vaginal fecal leakage.[31–33] In these cases, a rectovaginal fistula was thought to cause an infection and para-inflammatory state leading to SS, although 1 patient may have had underlying inflammatory bowel disease based on family history.[31–33] After 3 months of age, infectious etiologies are more common compared with the earlier neonatal period.[31] Immunodeficiency conditions found associated with neonatal SS include chronic granulomatous disease,[34] common variable immunodeficiency,[35,36] human immunodeficiency virus (HIV),[31] chronic atypical neutrophilic dermatosis with lipodystrophy and elevated temperature (CANDLE) syndrome with mutations in the PSMB8 gene,[31,37] and NFKB2 mutations.[38] Thus a referral to immunology or medical genetics may be appropriate, especially in patients with recurrent infections or in a family with known genetic disease. Importantly, when evaluating a patient with a possible underlying immunodeficiency, leukocytosis is not a reliable marker and, therefore, may be an irrelevant criterion in these patients.[13]

Grouping patients by age may help guide the clinical work-up because the frequency of these associations varies by age. Halpern and Salim[6] proposed separating patients into 2 age groups based on their risk of malignancy. Patients were categorized as younger than 3 years of age, termed as having infantile SS, and as 3 years to 18 years of age, termed as having junior SS.[6]

Table 1
Suggested workup for pediatric Sweet's syndrome

Diagnosis and Baseline	Obtain biopsy, tissue culture, CBC with differential, ESR, CRP, CMP, blood pressure, echocardiogram			
Associations	Neonatal SS (birth – less than 3 months)	Infantile SS (3 months – less than 3 yrs)	Junior SS (3 yrs - 18 yrs)	Workup[a]
Medication	Consider in all patients			Obtain drug history
IBD	Consider with symptoms and/or family history			Fecal calprotectin and referral to gastroenterology
Bone pain in context of possible infection, CRMO, or malignancy	Consider workup if presence of bone pain			Xray, and/or MRI
Infections	More common >3 months	Most common cause in this age group	Frequent cause	Workup guided by age and symptoms
Malignancy or paraneoplastic disorders	Consider workup, though not commonly reported in these age groups		Strongly recommend workup, frequent cause	LDH, uric acid, SPEP, and referral to hematology
Autoimmune or auto-inflammatory disease	Consider neonatal lupus, add EKG and maternal screening labs to workup	Consider with symptoms and family history		ANA, anti-SSA/Ro, anti-SSB/La, anti-U1RNP, anti-dsDNA, anti-RNP, anti-Smith, UA, and referral to rheumatology
Immunodeficiencies	More common <6 weeks	Less common > 6 months		Immunoglobulin levels, granulocyte and lymphocyte function tests, HIV testing, NBT, and referral to immunology/genetics

Rectovestibular Fistulas	Consider as a nidus of infection, para-inflammatory state, or sign of IBD		–	Physical exam and culture of drainage
Pregnancy	–	–	Consider workup in a pubescent female	Urine hCG

Abbreviations: ANA, antinuclear antibodies; ATRA, all-trans-retinoic acid; AZA, azathioprine; CBC, Complete blood cell count with differential; CMP, comprehensive metabolic panel; CRMO, chronic recurrent multifocal osteomyelitis; CRP, C-reactive protein; DISS, Drug induced Sweet's syndrome; ESR, erythrocyte sedimentation rate; G-CSF, Granulocyte colony-stimulating factor; hCG, human chorionic gonadotropin; HIV, human immunodeficiency virus; IBD, inflammatory bowel disease; LDH, lactate dehydrogenase; NBT, nitro blue tetrazolium test; SPEP, serum protein electrophoresis; SS, Sweet's Syndrome; TMP-SMX, trimethoprim-sulfamethoxazole.

[a] These are generalized guidelines based on available literature and workup should be guided by individual patient symptoms.

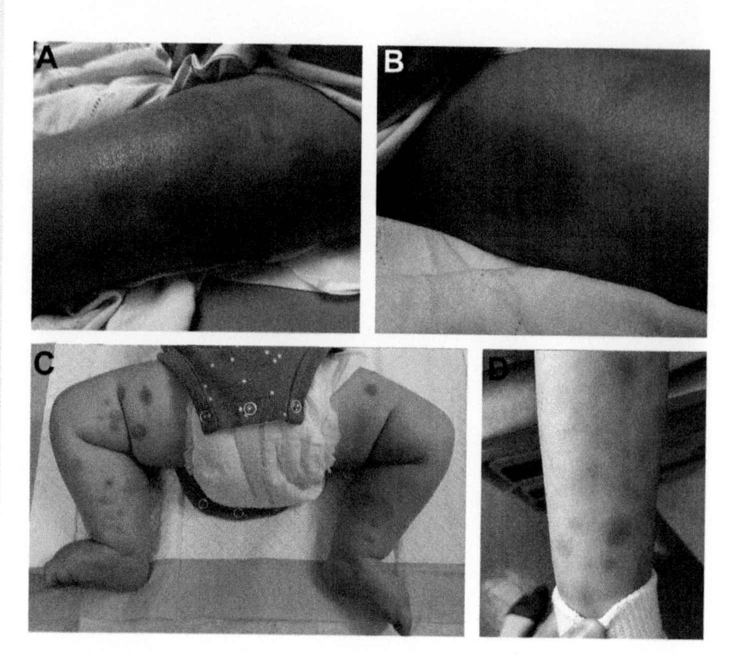

Fig. 1. Classic SS morphology on the (*A*) left thigh and (*B*) right thigh of a child with Hodgkin lymphoma, (*C*) in an infant with idiopathic SS, and (*D*) on a young girl with cystic fibrosis. (*A-D courtesy of* S. Leitenberger, MD, Portland, Oregon; B. Zimmerman, MD, Oakland, California; and J. Dhossche, MD, Portland, Oregon, respectively.)

Patients who are younger than 3 years old are more likely to be male and SS is more likely to be associated with infection.[8,39,40] Patients ages 3 years to 18 years demonstrate an equal male-to-female ratio, in comparison with adults, who are more commonly female.[6] Junior SS has an association with malignancy of approximately 44%, similar to adult SS.[6,31] The investigators note a paucity of cases of pediatric malignancy associated with pediatric SS in children under 3 years of age in the literature. It therefore is difficult to propose concrete screening guidelines for all pediatric SS patients.[6] Based on these differences within pediatric SS, the authors propose further separating patients into 3 groups: ages birth to age less than 3 months, termed as having neonatal SS; ages 3 months to less than 3 years, termed as having infantile SS; and ages 3 years to 18 years, termed as having junior SS (see **Table 1**).

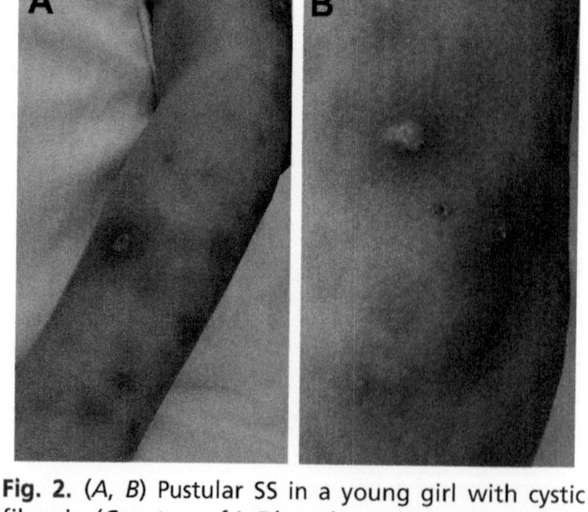

Fig. 2. (*A, B*) Pustular SS in a young girl with cystic fibrosis. (*Courtesy of* J. Dhossche, MD, Portland, OR)

Extracutaneous Manifestations

SS is associated with multiple extracutaneous manifestations.[11] Mucosal lesions are less common in children compared with adults.[1,6] Oral mucosal lesions often are associated with hematologic malignancies in adult patients but are found in only 5% of all pediatric SS patients and are not associated with malignancy specifically.[6] Conjunctivitis is associated more with the classic form of SS in this population.[41]

Cardiac complications from SS are associated most commonly with cases of cutis laxa.[6,25] The pathogenesis of cutis laxa is debated but thought to be due either to a deficiency in α-antitrypsin, allowing for increased destruction of dermal elastic tissues by proteases, or to inflammatory cells, releasing elastase.[42] The role of elastase in SS is suggested by the fact that dapsone is effective in treating swelling in the acute phase of acquired cutis laxa,[42] proposed to be due to its anti-inflammatory function of suppressing the release of elastase by neutrophils.[43] Cardiac complications, which can be silent and fatal, occur at variable time points following the initial diagnosis of pediatric SS. Some cases occur early, such as in the case of a 2 year old who developed SS and cutis laxa followed 16 days later by the development of heart failure, with ultimately a fatal

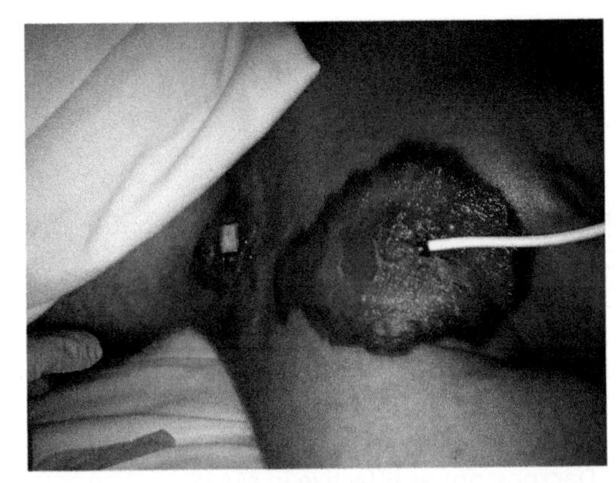

Fig. 3. Bullous SS in a child. (*Courtesy of* S. Leitenberger, MD, Portland, OR.)

outcome.[25] In comparison, some cardiac complications have occurred years later.[44,45] Aortitis and Takayasu arteritis have been reported approximately 4 years after SS diagnosis (with a range of 7 months to 8 years); 2 of these 5 cases had a fatal outcome.[46]

Approximately 5% of pediatric SS patients have pulmonary infiltrates on imaging.[6] Lung involvement is thought to be due to cytokine dysregulation and/or neutrophils releasing superoxide free radicals within the lung and can lead to the misdiagnosis of septic shock with fatal outcomes.[47] A rare, but severe, pulmonary manifestation has been described as bronchiolitis obliterans–like appearance/cryptogenic organizing pneumonia.[41] Most often pulmonary manifestations occur several months after cutaneous lesions but can present simultaneously or precede skin lesions, leading to a misdiagnosis or a delay in diagnosis.[41] For instance, 1 case of a patient with Fanconi anemia with severe progressive pneumonia unresponsive to antibiotics was found to have cutaneous SS 3 months later.[13,41]

Screening

Several recommended evaluations have been proposed by Lee and Chen[8] and Hospach and colleagues.[3] To fulfill the SS major criteria, skin biopsy usually is obtained. Tissue cultures (bacterial, mycobacterial, and fungal) often also are indicated. In some pediatric patients, a biopsy was not obtained when clinical suspicion for SS was high. For example, in a case of a patient with Fanconi anemia with poor wound healing, the authors deferred skin biopsy of SS lesions and proceeded with bone marrow biopsy, given their high suspicion for hematologic malignancy.[29] The authors encourage biopsy and cultures in all patients; however, individual variation in work-up may occur based on clinical context. To fulfill minor criteria, a complete blood cell count (CBC) with differential, C-reactive protein (CRP), erythrocyte sedimentation rate (ESR), and pregnancy test, when appropriate, should be obtained. Additionally, blood pressure and an echocardiogram should be obtained as baselines to follow and rule out cardiac complications/manifestations, described previously.[3] The suggested initial work-up for all patients can be found in **Table 1**.

Additional testing also has been recommended in the literature,[3,8] and the authors created a summary based on age and underlying association (see **Table 1**). A thorough drug history should be obtained for all patients. If a patient notes bone pain, Hospach and colleagues[3] recommended imaging with radiograph and then magnetic resonance imaging (MRI) if inconclusive or negative to evaluate for infection, CRMO, or malignancy. Referral to gastroenterology for evaluation of

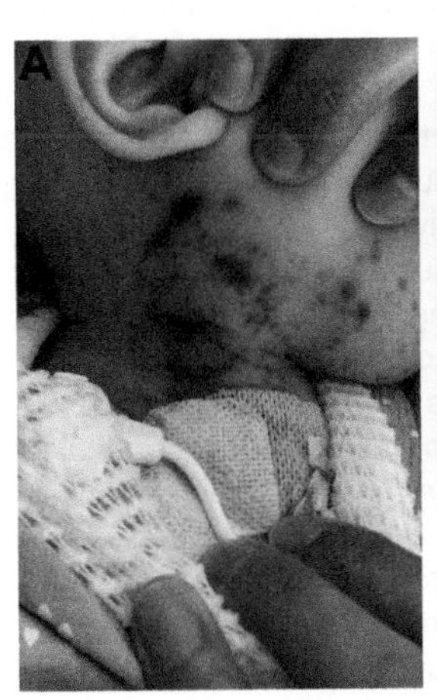

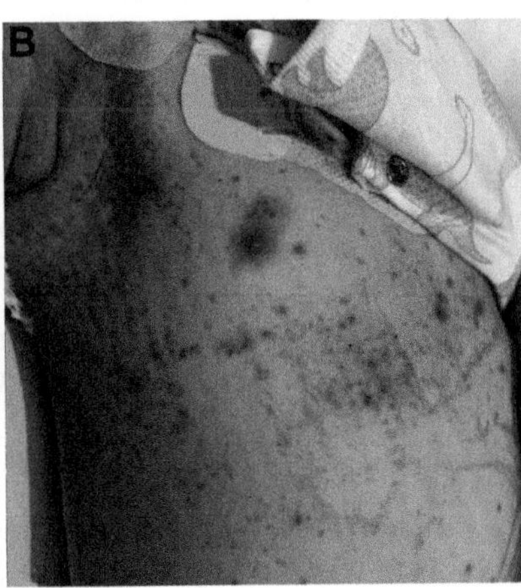

Fig. 4. An infant with acute myelogenous leukemia and thrombocytopenia presenting with (*A*) linear lesions demonstrating pathergy and (*B*) pustular and linear lesions. (*Courtesy of* B. Zimmerman, MD, Oakland, California.).

Table 2
Treatment of pediatric Sweet syndrome

Medication	Comments
First line[a]	
Systemic corticosteroids[5,11,24,55]	Recommend tapering over weeks to months
Local steroids (intralesional or topical)[11]	Consider for localized disease
SSKI[7,49]	Can be used as a steroid-sparing agent or to assist with tapering steroids
Colchicine[48]	Can be used as a steroid-sparing agent or to assist with tapering steroids
Second line[b]	
Dapsone ± IVIG[42,50]	• Dapsone not as effective in MASS • Dapsone effective in evolving cutis laxa to control swelling • Consider adding IVIG in the setting of immunodeficiency, especially if steroids contraindicated
Nonsteroidal anti-inflammatory drugs (indomethacin PR/PO)[7,23,56]	Refractory SS, HSS
Cyclosporine[5,7,56]	Refractory SS
TNF inhibitors (infliximab and etanercept)[3,24]	Refractory SS

[a] Should have excellent response to first-line therapies.
[b] Can be added to first-line treatments for improved tapering of first-line therapies.

inflammatory bowel disease is recommended with symptoms or a known family history. Infectious work-up should be age appropriate and include upper respiratory and gastrointestinal infections. Malignancies and paraneoplastic diseases, such as hematologic malignancies, Fanconi anemia, or aplastic anemia, can be screened with additional laboratory tests, referral to hematology/oncology, and consideration of bone marrow biopsy.[40] Autoimmune diseases can be evaluated based on symptoms or age, such as neonatal lupus in newborns, through a basic rheumatologic work-up and referral to rheumatology, when appropriate. Newborns may present with unique parainflammatory states in the context of malformations or fistulas, which may require special imaging and culturing of drainage, when present. Immunodeficiencies also should be considered in the neonatal period and can be evaluated with a basic immunologic work-up and referral to genetics/immunology.[31–33] Finally, pregnancy should be ruled out in pubescent female patients.

THERAPEUTIC OPTIONS

The primary treatment of SS is management of the underlying condition when identified. If DISS is suspected, withdrawal of the offending drug may resolve disease, although use of systemic corticosteroids may hasten resolution.[14] A summary of therapies can be found in **Table 2**. Clear dosing guidelines have not been established; however, references to individual reports of dosing are provided in **Table 2**.

First-line Therapies

First-line treatment of SS is corticosteroids, including prednisone or methylprednisolone pulse dosing.[5,11] Some investigators have used intralesional corticosteroid injections or high-potency topical steroids for localized SS.[11] Pediatric patients have recurrence of SS following steroid taper more often than adults,[2,5,8] leading to concern for long-term steroid use.[48] Steroid-sparing therapies often are necessary to mitigate the potential side effects of systemic corticosteroids.[2,48] Saturated solution of potassium iodide (SSKI) is highly effective for SS. According to Tangtatco and colleagues,[49] the recommended dosing for SSKI is 10 mg/kg/d to 40 mg/kg/d in 3 divided doses.[49] Adult dosing has been extrapolated to pediatric cases and described in the SS literature.[7,49] Investigators recommend continuing treatment until 6 weeks after clinical cure, followed by a slow taper based on clinical response. It is recommended to monitor thyroid function during and after treatment with SSKI.[49] Colchicine has been used for patients unable to taper off steroids or when SSKI is unsuccessful.[48]

Second-line Therapies

Second-line therapies in children include indomethacin, cyclosporine, and dapsone.[7] Dapsone is thought to be less effective in MASS[50]; however, it may be useful in treating evolving cutis laxa, as discussed previously.[42,51] The addition of intravenous immunoglobulin (IVIG) to dapsone has been used in immunodeficient children who do not respond well to standard treatments.[50] Other notable reported therapies include tumor necrosis factor (TNF) inhibitors (infliximab and etanercept), which have been used in some cases of refractory SS without a known association of inflammatory bowel disease (IBD).[3,24]

ONGOING MANAGEMENT

Ongoing dermatologic evaluation is important for monitoring active and recurrent cutaneous disease. Systemic disease can be subtle, and ongoing clinical, laboratory, and ancillary evaluation is important. Given the lack of data, long-term evaluation plans should be individualized.

Muster and colleagues[51] proposed clinical stages in SS, which may be beneficial in guiding management. These stages include an acute inflammatory stage, an intermediate stage with an evolving secondary cutis laxa with periodic acute exacerbations, and an inactive stage with postinflammatory cutis laxa and normal inflammatory laboratory values.[51] There have not been longitudinal studies following these patients through the different stages. How these stages correspond to long-term cardiac complications is unknown. Data also are lacking about whether closer cardiac monitoring is warranted for patients who are at higher risk for developing cutis laxa, such as those with pathergy. Due to the potentially fatal risk of cardiac complications, an individualized approach is important because a subset of patients may need increased monitoring. A thorough evaluation with echocardiogram and monitoring is important to evaluate for aortitis or aneurysm development in patients with acquired cutis laxa.[3] Hospach and colleagues[3] recommend echocardiography in patients with cutis laxa every 3 months into adulthood. Additionally, if any new-onset dyspnea appears after initial SS diagnosis, this could represent a cardiac or pulmonary manifestation, and evaluation is warranted.

TYING IT ALL TOGETHER: AN ILLUSTRATIVE CASE REPORT

We report a 3-year-old girl, who presented initially with 5 days of vomiting, diarrhea, fever (38.2°C), anorexia, rash, and mild leukocytosis of 19,000 cells/mm^3 (normal range 4.6–13.2 k/mm^3). COVID-19 testing was obtained and later found negative. A chest radiograph (CXR) was consistent with viral infection and/or reactive airway disease, with no focal consolidations. She was discharged when she improved clinically in the emergency department (ED).

One week later, she represented to the ED with a fever (38.5Co) and respiratory distress. She was intubated and admitted to the pediatric intensive care unit. On skin examination, there were 1-mm pustules coalescing on erythematous 1-cm to 4-cm plaques with violaceous, dusky centers on the abdomen, chest, back, and lower legs (**Fig. 5**). Her laboratory work-up was notable for a leukocytosis to 31,000 cells/mm^3 (normal range 4.6–13.2 k cells/mm^3), thrombocytosis to 495,000 platelets/mm^3 (normal range 189–394 k platelets/mm^3) and elevated lactic acid to 2.6 mmol/L (normal range 0.5–1.9 mmol/L), ESR

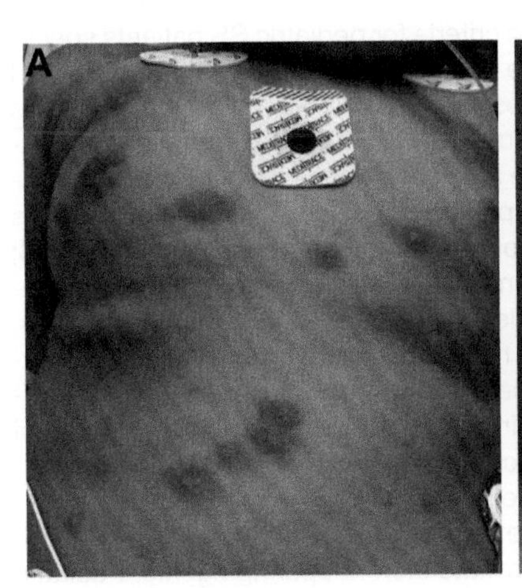

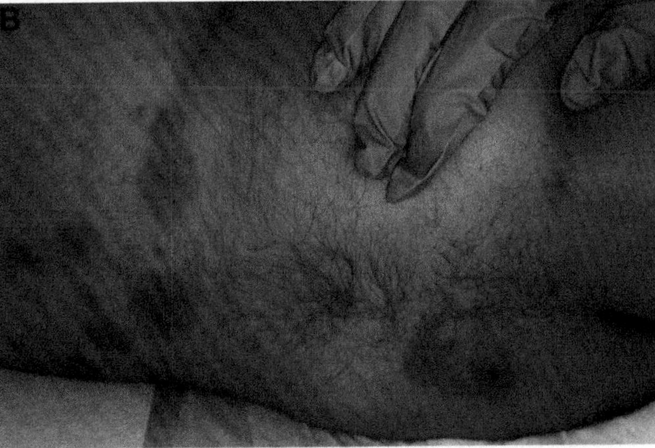

Fig. 5. (*A, B*) A 3-year-old girl with pustular SS in the setting of Crohn disease.

greater than 120 mm/h (normal range 0–20 mm/h), and CRP to 124 mg/L (normal range <10 mg/L). Computed tomography of the chest showed probable bacterial pneumonia with atelectasis. Pneumonia was suspected as the underlying diagnosis; however, an extensive infectious work-up, including respiratory panel, blood cultures, sputum cultures, throat cultures, tissue cultures, urine cultures, COVID-19 polymerase chain reaction (PCR), cytomegalovirus antibodies, Epstein-Barr virus panel, cryptococcal serum antigen, legionella urine antigen, herpes simplex virus/varicella zoster virus PCR, and broad-range PCR, all were negative. She improved and was extubated on hospital day 2. She continued to have intermittent fevers, and her inflammatory markers remained elevated, although down-trending. A skin biopsy showed a predominantly neutrophilic dermal infiltrate with subcorneal pustules and necrosis, leading to a clinicopathologic diagnosis of SS. A bone marrow biopsy showed no evidence of malignancy. Her condition improved and she was discharged home without a clear underlying association.

She presented to the ED for a third time approximately 4 weeks after her discharge with mouth ulcers and oral aversion. She was found to have diarrhea and complex aphthous stomatitis and was referred to pediatric gastroenterology. A fecal calprotectin was elevated to 2110 (<50 μg/g) and a colonoscopy demonstrated evidence of Crohn disease. Ultimately, her case was consistent with SS with severe pulmonary manifestations in the setting of inflammatory bowel disease. She has been treated with systemic steroids and transitioned to mercaptopurine and is doing well. This case highlights the diagnostic challenge of pulmonary SS, which often is mistaken for infection, delaying diagnosis and management. To the authors' knowledge, this is the first reported pediatric case of severe pulmonary SS requiring intubation in the setting of IBD, whereas pulmonary manifestations previously have been documented in the setting of malignancy or immunodeficiencies.[35,41,47]

DISCUSSION AND FUTURE DIRECTIONS

Pediatric SS patients have unique characteristics and considerations compared with adult SS patients. Pediatric patients thus far, however, have been diagnosed largely based on criteria that were created for adults.[9] In 1 report, only 50% of pediatric patients had a rash that was described as painful or tender, a major diagnostic criterion for SS; most had a leukocytosis (95%), elevated ESR (95%), and fever (85%).[6] It would be useful to understand further how effective the other diagnostic criteria are for capturing pediatric SS patients. Pediatric SS patients should be evaluated on a case-by-case basis, keeping the most likely underlying associations in mind and allowing these to guide work-up.

For patients under 3 months of age, immunodeficiencies and genetic syndromes should be considered as well as disorders specific to neonates, such as neonatal lupus erythematosus.[31] In patients ages 3 months to 3 years of age, infections are highly prevalent. In patients 3 years of age and older, malignancies occur at a similar prevalence to adult patients.[3] The authors attempt to review and summarize available literature and expand on previous distinctions based on age across all pediatric patients in order to help guide evaluation and ultimately management.

Without treatment, SS is thought to resolve over 1 month to 3 months in adults but may be more refractory in children, depending on the underlying etiology.[8] For instance, in neonatal lupus erythematous, patients have a good prognosis due to the resolution of the underlying inflammatory state, whereas those with a genetic or immunodeficiency syndrome may have a more prolonged course due to persistent inflammation and immune dysregulation.[31]

Although it is well established that SS represents a hypersensitivity reaction to an inflammatory state, not much is known about the pathophysiology. Cases of genetic or familial SS may help further the understanding of the pathophysiology of SS.[52,53] Other studies have proposed associations with HLA in the development of SS.[15,33,54] The cytokine signature of SS likely is complex and hard to generalize but could offer insights for personalized care.[48]

SUMMARY

Diagnostic criteria for pediatric SS patients specifically have not been established. Having defined age groups in pediatric SS may help clinicians guide evaluation and management of pediatric patients. The authors propose further separating pediatric SS patients into 3 groups: ages birth to less than 3 months, termed as having neonatal SS; ages 3 months to less than 3 years, termed as having infantile SS; and ages 3 years to 18 years, termed as having junior SS. Identifying an underlying disease association, when present, is important for directed treatment and management of potential complications. Although pediatric patients have excellent response to steroids, they have more recurrence after steroid taper, which may necessitate steroid-sparing agents. Pediatric SS patients are at risk for severe extracutaneous manifestations. Data are lacking in pediatric SS and more studies are needed to better understand the pathophysiology and long-term management of the disorder.

CLINICS CARE POINTS

- All patients with suspected SS should have basic evaluation to identify typical triggers, with directed work-up based on patient age, signs, and symptoms.
- Pediatric SS typically has great response to first-line therapies, although, due to multiple recurrences, may depend on second-line therapies to taper off steroids successfully.
- Pediatric SS patients are at risk for severe extracutaneous manifestations and need long-term monitoring.

DISCLOSURE

The authors have nothing to disclose.

REFERENCES

1. Sweet RB. An acute febrile neutrophtlic dermatosts. Br J Dermatol 1964;76(8–9):349–56.
2. Herron MD, Coffin CM, Vanderhooft SL. Sweet syndrome in two children. Pediatr Dermatol 2005; 22(6):525–9.
3. Hospach T, von den Driesch P, Dannecker GE. Acute febrile neutrophilic dermatosis (Sweet's syndrome) in childhood and adolescence: two new patients and review of the literature on associated diseases. Eur J Pediatr 2009;168(1):1–9.
4. García-Romero MT, Ho N. Pediatric Sweet syndrome. A retrospective study. Int J Dermatol 2015; 54(5):518–22.
5. Uihlein LC, Brandling-Bennett HA, Lio PA, et al. Sweet syndrome in children. Pediatr Dermatol 2012;29(1):38–44.
6. Halpern J, Salim A. Pediatric sweet syndrome: case report and literature review. Pediatr Dermatol 2009; 26(4):452–7.
7. Cohen PR. Sweet's syndrome – a comprehensive review of an acute febrile neutrophilic dermatosis. Orphanet J Rare Dis 2007;2(1):34.
8. Lee GL, Chen AY-Y. Neutrophilic dermatoses: Kids are not just little people. Clin Dermatol 2017;35(6): 541–54.
9. von den Driesch P. Sweet's syndrome (acute febrile neutrophilic dermatosis). J Am Acad Dermatol 1994; 31(4):535–56.
10. Anzalone CL, Cohen PR. Acute febrile neutrophilic dermatosis (Sweet's syndrome). Curr Opin Hematol 2013;20(1):26–35.
11. Cohen PR. Neutrophilic dermatoses: a review of current treatment options. Am J Clin Dermatol 2009; 10(5):301–12.
12. Su WP, Liu HN. Diagnostic criteria for Sweet's syndrome. Cutis 1986;37(3):167–74.
13. Chatham-Stephens K, Devere T, Guzman-Cottrill J, et al. Metachronous manifestations of Sweet's syndrome in a neutropenic patient with Fanconi anemia. Pediatr Blood Cancer 2008;51(1):128–30.
14. Cohen PR, Kurzrock R. Sweet's syndrome revisited: a review of disease concepts. Int J Dermatol 2003; 42(10):761–78.
15. Stevens GJ, Yutronic HJ, Pizarro OJ, et al. Sweet syndrome in pediatrics. A case report. Rev Chil Pediatr 2018;89(4):511–5.
16. Walker DC, Cohen PR. Trimethoprim-sulfamethoxazole-associated acute febrile neutrophilic dermatosis: Case report and review of drug-induced Sweet's syndrome. J Am Acad Dermatol 1996; 34(5):918–23.
17. Kim MJ, Choe YH. EPONYM. Sweet syndrome. Eur J Pediatr 2010;169(12):1439–44.
18. Kim MJ, Jang KT, Choe YH. Azathioprine hypersensitivity presenting as sweet syndrome in a child with ulcerative colitis. Indian Pediatr 2011;48:3.
19. Fernández-Torres RM, Castro S, Moreno A, et al. Subcutaneous histiocytoid sweet syndrome associated with crohn disease in an adolescent. Case Rep Dermatol Med 2014;2014:954254.
20. Kim J, Seo J, Oh SH. Unusual presentation of histiocytoid Sweet's syndrome in a pediatric patient. Int J Dermatol 2015;54(12):e555–7.
21. Camarillo D, McCalmont TH, Frieden IJ, et al. Two pediatric cases of nonbullous histiocytoid neutrophilic dermatitis presenting as a cutaneous manifestation of lupus erythematosus. Arch Dermatol 2008; 144(11):1495–8.
22. Peroni A, Colato C, Schena D, et al. Histiocytoid Sweet syndrome is infiltrated predominantly by M2-like macrophages. J Am Acad Dermatol 2015; 72(1):131–9.
23. Yeom SD, Ko HS, Moon JH, et al. Histiocytoid Sweet Syndrome in a Child without Underlying Systemic Disease. Ann Dermatol 2017;29(5):626–9.
24. Knöpfel N, Theiler M, Luchsinger I, et al. Infliximab for the treatment of recalcitrant bullous Sweet syndrome in a 10-year-old girl. Pediatr Dermatol 2020. https://doi.org/10.1111/pde.14356.
25. Guhamajumdar M, Agarwala B. Sweet syndrome, cutis laxa, and fatal cardiac manifestations in a 2-year-old girl. Tex Heart Inst J 2011;38(3):285–7.
26. Chen S-H, Kuo Y-T, Liu Y-L, et al. Acute myeloid leukemia presenting with sweet syndrome: a case

report and review of the literature. Pediatr Neonatol 2017;58(3):283–4.
27. Bucchia M, Barbarot S, Reumaux H, et al. Age-specific characteristics of neutrophilic dermatoses and neutrophilic diseases in children. J Eur Acad Dermatol Venereol 2019;33(11):2179–87.
28. Abbas O, Kibbi A-G, Rubeiz N. Sweet's syndrome: retrospective study of clinical and histologic features of 44 cases from a tertiary care center. Int J Dermatol 2010;49(11):1244–9.
29. Webber L, Cummins M, Mann R, et al. Panniculitis in a 3-year-old child with Fanconi anemia-associated bone marrow hypoplasia heralds transformation to acute myeloid leukemia. Pediatr Dermatol 2019; 36(5):725–7.
30. Barton JL, Pincus L, Yazdany J, et al. Association of sweet's syndrome and systemic lupus erythematosus. Case Rep Rheumatol 2011;2011:242681.
31. Gray PEA, Bock V, Ziegler DS, et al. Neonatal sweet syndrome: a potential marker of serious systemic illness. Pediatrics 2012;129(5):e1353–9.
32. Shinozuka J, Tomiyama H, Tanaka S-I, et al. Neonatal sweet's syndrome associated with rectovestibular fistula with normal anus. Pediatr Rep 2015;7(2):5858.
33. Omoya K, Naiki Y, Kato Z, et al. Sweet's syndrome in a neonate with non-B54 types of human leukocyte antigen. World J Pediatr 2012;8(2):181–4.
34. Knipstein JA, Ambruso DR. Sweet syndrome in an infant with chronic granulomatous disease. J Pediatr Hematol Oncol 2012;34(5):372–4.
35. Cook QS, Zdanski CJ, Burkhart CN, et al. Idiopathic, refractory sweet's syndrome associated with common variable immunodeficiency: a case report and literature review. Curr Allergy Asthma Rep 2019; 19(6):32.
36. O'Regan GM, Kemperman PM, Sandilands A, et al. Raman profiles of the stratum corneum define 3 filaggrin genotype-determined atopic dermatitis endophenotypes. J Allergy Clin Immunol 2010;126:574–80.e1.
37. Liu Y, Ramot Y, Torrelo A, et al. Mutations in proteasome subunit β type 8 cause chronic atypical neutrophilic dermatosis with lipodystrophy and elevated temperature with evidence of genetic and phenotypic heterogeneity: Mutations in *PSMB8* Cause Candle Syndrome. Arthritis Rheum 2012; 64(3):895–907.
38. Okamura K, Uchida T, Hayashi M, et al. Neutrophilic dermatosis associated with an NFKB2 mutation. Clin Exp Dermatol 2019;44(3):350–2.
39. Warren JT, Miller CP, White AJ. 7-Year-Old With a Painful Rash. JAMA Pediatr 2016;170(8):801–2.
40. Hsieh J, Yalcindag A, Coghlin DT. A Sweet Case of Mycoplasma. Pediatrics 2017;140(3). https://doi.org/10.1542/peds.2016-2762.
41. Tzelepis E, Kampolis CF, Vlachadami I, et al. Cryptogenic organizing pneumonia in Sweet's syndrome: case report and review of the literature. Clin Respir J 2016;10(2):250–4.
42. Fontenelle E, Almeida APM de, Souza GMA de A. Marshall's syndrome. An Bras Dermatol 2013; 88(2):279–82.
43. Suda T, Suzuki Y, Matsui T, et al. Dapsone suppresses human neutrophil superoxide production and elastase release in a calcium-dependent manner. Br J Dermatol 2005;152(5):887–95.
44. Guia JM, Frias J, Castro FJ, et al. Cardiovascular involvement in a boy with Sweet's syndrome. Pediatr Cardiol 1999;20(4):295–7.
45. Stos B, Hatchuel Y, Bonnet D. Mitral valvar regurgitation in a child with Sweet's syndrome. Cardiol Young 2007;17(2):218–9.
46. Ma EH, Akikusa JD, MacGregor D, et al. Sweet's syndrome with postinflammatory elastolysis and Takayasu arteritis in a child: a case report and literature review. Pediatr Dermatol 2012;29(5):645–50.
47. Kinser KN, Panach K, Dominguez AR. Recurrent Malignancy-Associated Atypical Neutrophilic Dermatosis With Noninfectious Shock. Am J Med Sci 2017;354(6):626–32.
48. Takano Y, Fujino H, Yachie A, et al. Serum cytokine profile in pediatric Sweet's syndrome: a case report. J Med Case Rep 2017;11(1):178.
49. Tangtatco JAA, Ho N, Drucker A, et al. Potassium iodide in refractory, recurrent pediatric Sweet syndrome: Guidance in dosing and monitoring. Pediatr Dermatol 2018;35(2):271–3.
50. Haliasos E, Soder B, Rubenstein DS, et al. Pediatric sweet syndrome and immunodeficiency successfully treated with intravenous immunoglobulin. Pediatr Dermatol 2005;22(6):530–5.
51. Muster AJ, Bharati S, Herman JJ, et al. Fatal cardiovascular disease and cutis laxa following acute febrile neutrophilic dermatosis. J Pediatr 1983; 102(2):243–8.
52. Parsapour K, Reep MD, Gohar K, et al. Familial sweet's syndrome in 2 brothers, both seen in the first 2 weeks of life. J Am Acad Dermatol 2003;49(1): 132–8.
53. Oskay T, Anadolu R. Sweet's syndrome in familial Mediterranean fever: possible continuum of the neutrophilic reaction as a new cutaneous feature of FMF. J Cutan Pathol 2009;36(8):901–5.
54. Mizoguchi M. Human Leukocyte Antigen in Sweet's Syndrome and Its Relationship to Behçet's Disease. Arch Dermatol 1988;124(7):1069.
55. Assari R, Ziaee V, Parvaneh N, et al. Periodic fever and neutrophilic dermatosis: is it sweet's syndrome? Case Rep Immunol 2014;2014:320920.
56. Sfrijan D, Visan SM, Zurac S, Diaconu B, Scurtu C. A Case of Sweet's Syndrome Secondary to Myelodysplastic Syndrome – Diagnostic and Treatment Challenges. Maedica (Bucur) 2016;11(2):154–7.

Morbilliform Eruptions in the Hospitalized Child

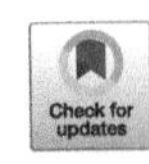

Jessica S. Haber, MD[a], Sarah D. Cipriano, MD, MPH, MS[b], Vikash S. Oza, MD[a,*]

KEYWORDS

- Morbilliform eruption • Pediatric • Inpatient dermatology • Diagnosis • Management
- Viral exanthem • Drug eruption

KEY POINTS

- Morbilliform eruptions are common in the pediatric inpatient setting.
- Accurate diagnosis relies on a thorough full-body physical examination and complete history.
- Infectious causes, such as measles, arboviridae, and Rocky Mountain spotted fever, should be considered in patients with morbilliform eruption and the appropriate vaccination and travel history.
- Both simple and complex drug eruptions can present with a morbilliform morphology in the hospitalized child and must be differentiated.
- Other inflammatory conditions, such as Kawasaki disease, and in the COVID-19 era, multisystem inflammatory syndrome in children, should be on a differential diagnosis of a child with fever and morbilliform eruption.
- Graft-versus-host disease and engraftment syndrome are 2 causes of morbilliform eruption that should be considered in the child with a transplant.

MORBILLIFORM ERUPTIONS IN THE HOSPITALIZED CHILD

The ability to accurately diagnose a child with a new-onset eruption in a timely manner is a fundamental skill for the dermatology consultant. Morbilliform eruptions inspire a broad and varied differential spanning across inflammatory and infectious categories. The goal of this article is to help the clinician develop an approach toward the pediatric patient with a morbilliform eruption in the emergency room or hospital setting. The authors review several high-yield clinical scenarios with a focus on recently emerging and reemerging childhood diagnoses.

THE HISTORY AND DEFINITION OF THE MORBILLIFORM ERUPTION

The term morbilliform originates from *morbilli*, the Italian diminutive of Il Morbo. In the Middle Ages, Il Morbo, or the great plague, referred to smallpox, and *morbilli* described the "small plague" of measles, as both epidemics have cooccurred since the sixth century.[1,2] Over time, the term morbilliform has been adopted to describe any eruption resembling measles. By definition, a morbilliform eruption is generalized and symmetric with involvement of the trunk and some portion of the extremities. The primary morphology is blanching, erythematous pink to red macules and papules that become confluent with time (**Fig. 1**). Today, morbilliform is a descriptor well engrained in the dermatology lexicon, often used synonymously with maculopapular exanthem, and defines eruptions that are distinct from those that are urticarial, eczematous, psoriasiform, pustular, vesicular, or vasculitic.

EVALUATION OF THE CHILD WITH A MORBILLIFORM ERUPTION

A fever and morbilliform eruption in a child should prompt a thorough evaluation for either an

[a] Ronald O. Perelman Department of Dermatology, NYU Grossman School of Medicine, NYU Langone Dermatology Associates, 240 East 38th Street, 12th Floor, New York, NY 10016, USA; [b] Department of Dermatology, University of Utah, 81 North Mario Capecchi Drive, Salt Lake City, UT 84113, USA
* Corresponding author.
E-mail address: Vikash.Oza@nyulangone.org

Dermatol Clin 40 (2022) 191–202
https://doi.org/10.1016/j.det.2021.12.006
0733-8635/22/© 2021 Elsevier Inc. All rights reserved.

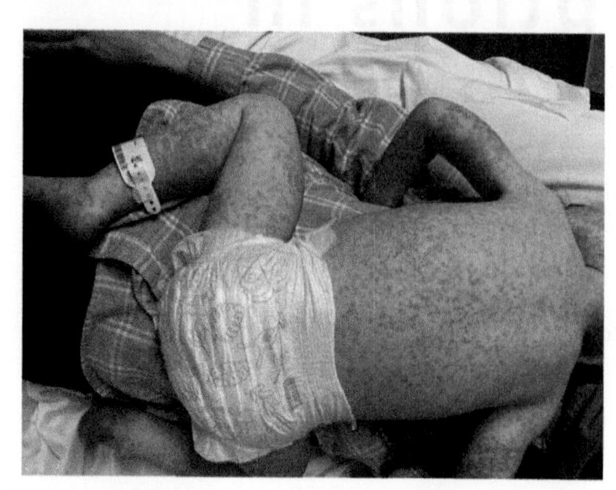

Fig. 1. Morbilliform eruption. A young child with acute Epstein-Barr virus infection with associated morbilliform rash.

infection, a medication allergy, or other systemic illness (eg, Kawasaki disease). Commonly implicated infections include enterovirus, adenovirus, Herpesviridae (Epstein-Barr virus, human cytomegalovirus, and human herpes virus 6 [HHV-6]), and parvovirus. Other respiratory infections, such as influenza B and *Mycoplasma pneumoniae*, may also cause morbilliform eruptions.[3] Because morbilliform eruptions can also be harbingers of more serious illness, the physician's task is to integrate an illness's timeline, a child's past medical history, exposures, and recent public health trends to ensure a comprehensive evaluation.

History Taking

The history should focus on a child's exposures (relevant sick contacts, a detailed travel history, infections circulating in the community, and medications) and their own host risk factors (vaccination and immune system status). Because morbilliform eruptions indicate a systemic inflammatory response, a complete review of systems should always be obtained.

Physical Examination

A full-body skin examination is necessary in all cases. Caregiver-provided photographs can be invaluable in illustrating the progression of a rash and in deciphering more subtle clinical findings, such as swelling. The conjunctiva, oral mucosa, genitalia, palms, soles, and lymph nodes should not be overlooked on the physical examination. Attention should also be paid to how an eruption has progressed. Certain eruptions, such as measles and drug rash with eosinophilia and systemic symptoms (DRESS), have facial involvement early in the course. Last, in an ill child with fever and a morbilliform eruption, the findings of petechiae and purpura serve as red flags for potentially life-threatening illnesses, such as Rocky Mountain spotted fever (RMSF), meningococcemia, or evolving disseminated intravascular coagulation.

Laboratory Evaluation

The laboratory workup is dictated by the differential diagnosis being considered (**Table 1**).

Management

Treatment should focus on the underlying illness. For patients who have symptoms related to their morbilliform eruption, low- to medium-strength topical corticosteroids can help.

MORBILLIFORM ERUPTIONS IN THE UNVACCINATED CHILD

Before widespread childhood vaccination, measles and rubella (also known as German measles or 3-day measles) were the primary cause of morbilliform eruptions in children. In the early twentieth century, more than 500,000 cases of measles (rubeola) were reported in the United States each year.[4,5] By 2000, the World Health Organization declared measles eliminated in the US, a historic achievement resulting from the measles vaccine introduced in 1963.[6]

Unfortunately, measles is still a common cause of childhood morbidity and mortality globally, especially within Africa and India, and rates are surging with a 50% increase in mortality since 2016.[7] Over the past decade, multiple outbreaks have occurred in the United States, with the convergence of imported cases from travel, and their spread within undervaccinated or unvaccinated populations. The largest outbreak occurred in 2019 with 1249 cases reported across 31 states.[8] The outbreak's epicenter was close-knit Orthodox Jewish communities within New York City, which accounted for 75% of the cases. Within this outbreak, the median age of patients was 5 year old, and 71% were unvaccinated.[8] The recent severe acute respiratory syndrome coronavirus 2 (SARS-CoV-2; COVID-19) pandemic has heightened concerns of a measles resurgence because of the disruption of well-child visits and vaccinations. A study in Alabama found overall vaccination rates to have declined by 10% from 2019 to 2020, and a reduction in measles, mumps, and rubella (MMR) vaccination by 54.7% over the same time period.[9]

For the clinician evaluating a child with fever and morbilliform eruption, accurate documentation of a child's vaccine status and travel history is critical. In the setting of an outbreak, children under

Table 1
Confirmatory testing for select infectious causes of morbilliform eruptions in children

Diagnosis	Laboratory Workup
Measles	Measles-specific IgM and RT-PCR from throat or nasal swab
Zika	RT-PCR of serum and urine for Zika RNA if ≤7 d of illness Zika-specific IgM positive if >7 d of illness (IgM can remain positive for months to years and can cross-react with Dengue)
Chikungunya	RT-PCR of serum if ≤ 7d of illness Chikungunya-specific IgM if >7 d since onset of illness
Dengue	RT-PCR of serum if ≤7 d of illness Dengue-specific IgM if >7 d since onset of illness
RMSF	Diagnosis can rarely be established during the early phase so empiric treatment should be started Convalescent antibody titer through indirect immunofluorescence antibody testing for IgG against the *R rickettsii* antigen

the age of 5 are the most vulnerable because of incomplete vaccination with the MMR vaccine being administered typically at 1 and 4 to 5 years of age.[10] Measles is a highly transmissible, airborne virus with an attack rate of 90% in susceptible, exposed individuals.[11] Therefore, any consideration for measles should immediately prompt isolation and airborne precautions. Children with measles present with a prodrome lasting 2 to 4 days consisting of fever up to 104°F and the classic 3 C's of cough, coryza (rhinitis), and conjunctivitis. The pathognomonic enanthem, Koplik spots, consists of clustered gray-white to pink papules located on the buccal mucosa (**Fig. 2**). Koplik spots may be absent at the time of dermatologic evaluation because their onset precedes the exanthem by 48 hours and only lasts 12 to 72 hours.[12,13] Classically, the exanthem starts 2 to 4 days after the prodrome, lasts 6 to 7 days, and spreads in a cephalocaudal pattern beginning on the face, favoring the forehead, hairline, and posterior auricular area. Many routine childhood exanthems instead start on the trunk and typically spare the face. As the exanthem progresses, it fades in the order that it appeared and can adopt a brownish discoloration in lighter-skinned patients. Measles has an incubation period of 10 days, and patients are contagious 5 days before the onset of the rash and for 4 days after its disappearance.[13] A child suspected of having measles should have both a serum measles-specific immunoglobulin M (IgM) antibody test and a respiratory real-time polymerase chain reaction (RT-PCR) test from a throat or nasopharyngeal swab performed.[14] Children hospitalized for measles should receive supportive care. Administration of vitamin A and ribavirin may have a role in severe cases.[15]

MORBILLIFORM ERUPTIONS IN THE RETURNING TRAVELER

Travel screening has increasingly become a routine component of triage in pediatric emergency departments because of public health concerns over emerging infections, such as Ebola, Zika, and now

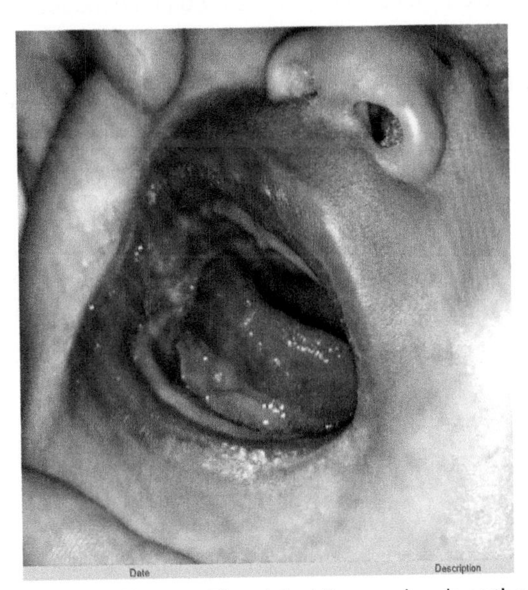

Fig. 2. Koplik spots. Pinpoint white macules along the buccal mucosa in an infant with measles infection.

COVID-19.[16] In addition to asking about any travel within the past 21 days, a detailed travel history also includes other relevant information to help narrow the differential. In the child with a fever and rash, important considerations include arboviruses (Zika, Dengue, Chikungunya), Brucellosis, Leptospirosis, Rickettsial diseases, and again, measles, depending on a child's vaccination status. In light of this, a travel history should document purpose of travel (tourist, visiting family and friends), location (urban vs rural), mosquito bites (arboviruses), tick bites (rickettsial diseases), exposure to unpasteurized dairy products (brucellosis), livestock exposure (leptospirosis), and freshwater exposure (leptospirosis). The article focuses on the arboviruses Zika, Dengue, and Chikungunya and the rickettsial infection RMSF, as the incidence of these infections is on the increase.[17,18]

Zika, Dengue, and Chikungunya are endemic in parts of the Caribbean, Central America, and South America.[19] The main vector for these viruses is the *Aedes aegypti* and *Aedes albopictus* mosquitoes. Several factors linked to their continued geographic spread include global warming, travel, and urbanization.[20] All 3 arboviruses have considerable overlap and should be considered when a child presents with fever, rash, conjunctivitis, and/or arthralgia after travel (**Table 2**).

Zika (Equatorial Africa and Asia, Pacific Islands, Caribbean, Latin America, North America)

Zika virus (ZIKV) is a *flavivirus* predominantly transmitted by mosquitos, with less common modes of transmission being sexual, intrauterine, perinatal, and laboratory exposure. From 2015 to 2016, a large outbreak of ZIKV occurred within the Americas, resulting in travel-associated cases in the United States but also local transmission in Florida and Texas.[21] As of 2020, no confirmed cases of ZIKV have been reported in the United States.[22] Eighty percent of cases are asymptomatic. The incubation period of Zika lasts from 3 to 14 days.[19] Acute infection is typically mild with rash, low-grade fever, arthralgia, myalgias, and nonpurulent conjunctivitis. Rash is common and was documented in 90% of patients in 1 cohort with ZIKV.[23] The ZIKV exanthem has been described as "distinct papules" descending from the trunk to the lower body, which can involve the palms and soles.[24] Mucosal involvement includes conjunctivitis and palatal petechiae.[24] Although acute infection is often self-limited, complications can include Guillain-Barre syndrome and congenital Zika syndrome from vertical transmission during pregnancy, leading to cerebral calcifications, severe microcephaly, intrauterine growth restriction, congenital contractures, ophthalmologic disease, and potentially fetal demise.[25,26]

Chikungunya (Asia, Africa, Latin America, Caribbean, Florida, Puerto Rico, US Virgin Islands)

Chikengunya virus (CHIKV) of the Togaviridae family has an expanding geographic spread.[27] Since 2013, CHIKV has expanded to include the Americas, particularly the Dominican Republic, Puerto Rico, and Haiti.[28] The incubation period can vary between 1 and 12 days.[19] Acute infection is

Table 2
Mucocutaneous characteristics of arbovirus infections

	Zika	Chikungunya	Dengue
Incubation period, d	3–14	1–12	5–8
Cutaneous manifestations in symptomatic individuals	90% of infections, morbilliform or fine papular eruption, descends from trunk to lower extremities, can be pruritic	~50% of infections, morbilliform, typically *spares face*, involves trunk and limbs, can be pruritic *Chik sign: centrofacial hyperpigmentation*	~50% of infections, *facial*, trunk, extremities, white "islands in sea of red," confluent erythema that can progress to morbilliform, typically not pruritic, usually spares palms and soles
Mucosal findings	Common, 55%, nonpurulent conjunctivitis	Uncommon	–15% to 30%, conjunctival or scleral injection, cracked lips, strawberry tongue, vesicles on soft palate
Laboratory findings	Nonspecific	Nonspecific	Thrombocytopenia

characterized by a high fever for 3 to 5 days, arthralgias, myalgias, and rash. As CHIKV can replicate within joint spaces, polyarthralgia is a hallmark feature and can occur before the onset of fever.[29] A maculopapular eruption occurs in 50% of cases, involving the trunk and extremities, occasionally the palms and soles, and appears 2 to 5 days after the fever starts.[8,19,30] It classically spares the face and can have islands of sparing similar to Dengue.[31] The rash resolves within 7 to 10 days of onset, whereas arthritis and arthralgias can persist for up to 3 years.[29] The "Chik sign" refers to postinfectious, centrofacial hyperpigmentation with a predilection for the nose and is well documented in children[31] (**Fig. 3**).

Dengue (Tropics and Subtropics)

Dengue is a mosquito-borne *flavivirus* endemic in popular tourist destinations in the Caribbean, Central and South America, Southeast Asia, Africa, and the Pacific Islands. Dengue ranges from being asymptomatic (75% of cases) to a life-threatening disease.[32] The incubation period ranges from 5 to 8 days following a bite from a mosquito with a high viral load. Classic dengue consists of fevers lasting 2 to 5 days, retro-orbital pain, nausea, vomiting, myalgia, arthralgias, and a morbilliform rash.[33] The rash of Dengue occurs in approximately 50% of symptomatic infections and within the first 24 to 48 hours of the illness.[19,34] Often referred to as "white islands in a sea of red," the Dengue exanthem has unaffected skin interspersed among broad patches of erythema[34] (**Fig. 4**). The febrile phase can be followed by either a defervescence phase, whereby the patient recovers, or Dengue hemorrhagic fever (DHF), characterized by increased vascular permeability, plasma leakage, and subsequent volume depletion.[33] DHF typically occurs in patients who have been previously infected and are then reinfected with a different viral strain. DHF more often affects children less than 15 years of age and has a more severe course, including facial flushing, vomiting, circumoral pallor, and cyanosis.[35] Petechiae, purpura, or ecchymoses can also be seen because of hemorrhage and are typically a sign of more severe forms of the disease, such as DHF or Dengue septic shock.[19,34] Mucosal involvement is also more common with DHF than with dengue fever, occurring in 15% to 30%, and can include conjunctival and scleral injection, cracked lips, strawberry tongue, and vesicles on the soft palate.[34] Most individuals develop thrombocytopenia, which can result in severe bleeding.[19] Diagnosis can be confirmed by viral serologic testing and by both PCR and enzyme-

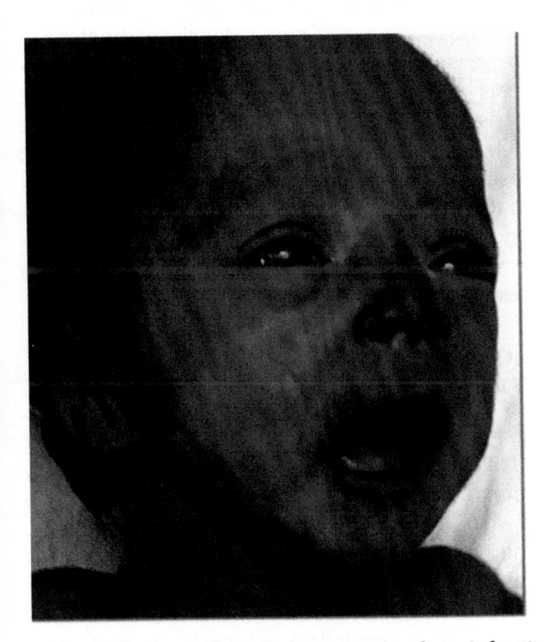

Fig. 3. Chik sign. Clinical photograph of an infant's face demonstrates a positive chik sign. (*From* Dabas G, Vinay K, Mahajan R. Diffuse Hyperpigmentation in Infants During Monsoon Season. JAMA Dermatol. 2020 Jan 1;156(1):99-101.)

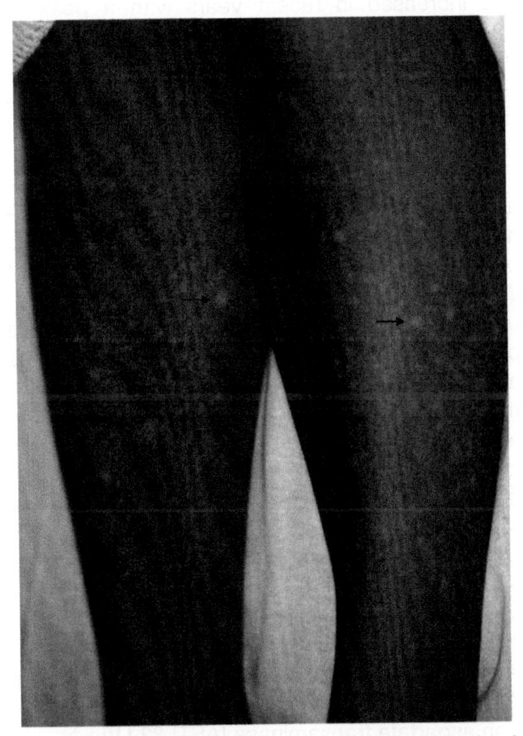

Fig. 4. Dengue virus. Pinpoint petechiae and islands of sparing (*arrows*) on a background of erythema. (*From* Pincus LB, Grossman ME, Fox LP. The exanthem of dengue fever: Clinical features of two US tourists traveling abroad. J Am Acad Dermatol. 2008 Feb;58(2):308-16.)

linked immunosorbent assay for RNA and dengue viral protein, respectively.[36]

RICKETTSIAL DISEASES: ROCKY MOUNTAIN SPOTTED FEVER

Paralleling the increase in arboviruses, tick-borne illnesses within the United States have also seen an increase in incidence and geographic spread.[37] RMSF is one of the most lethal tick-borne illnesses, and clinicians must maintain a high index of suspicion when evaluating a child with a fever and rash whether they practice in an endemic area or not. RMSF is caused by *Rickettsia rickettsii*, an obligate, intracellular bacteria transmitted by the dog tick (*Dermacentor variabilis*) in the Eastern United States and wood tick (*Dermacentor andersoni*) in the Western United States and Canada.[38] RMSF has also been documented in central Mexico, Panama, Costa Rica, northwestern Argentina, Brazil, and Columbia.[39] More than half of the cases in the United States originate from North Carolina, South Carolina, Tennessee, Oklahoma, and Arkansas; however, cases have been found in all 48 contiguous states except for Maine and Vermont.[40] The incidence of RMSF has increased in recent years with a peak of 6248 cases reported in 2017.[41] RMSF preferentially afflicts children less than 10 years old and adults 40 to 64 years of age.[42] Transmission is highest during the spring and summer months of April to August.[38]

Classically, RMSF presents with fever, headache, and rash, but the complete triad is uncommon.[38] An exanthem is seen in 97% of pediatric patients typically starting within the first 2 days of illness onset.[43] Small, 1- to 5-mm blanching macules typically begin on the wrists and ankles and progress to involve the palms and soles, arms and legs, and then trunk (**Fig. 5**). By the end of the first week, a morbilliform eruption often admixed with petechiae is seen.[44] However, it is crucial not to anchor the diagnosis on the finding of petechiae. In a case series of 92 children, 32% never developed a petechial component.[43] Other clinical and laboratory findings supportive of a diagnosis of RMSF and found in greater 50% of children include nausea and vomiting, thrombocytopenia (platelets <150,000/mm^3), hyponatremia (<135 mEq/dL), and transaminitis (median alanine transaminase [ALT] 55 U/L, median aspartate transaminase [AST] 83 U/L).[43]

Because RMSF can be fatal if treatment is delayed beyond the first 5 days of illness, treatment should be started as soon as the diagnosis is entertained.[45,46] Doxycycline is the first-line treatment irrespective of a child's age, as advised

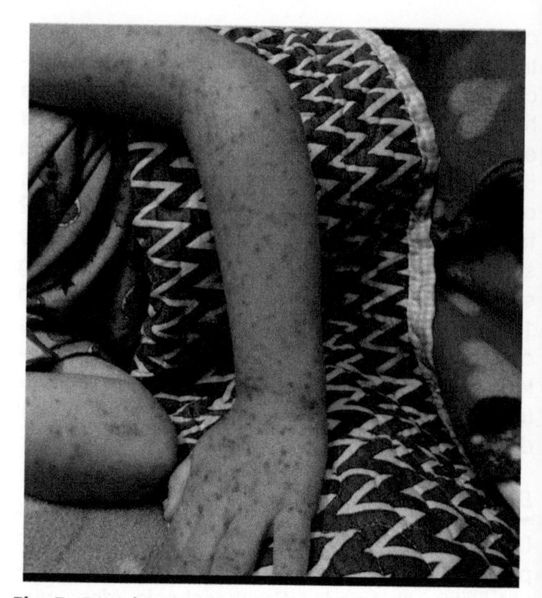

Fig. 5. Petechiae and purpuric macules in a child with RMSF.

by both the Centers for Disease Control and Prevention and the American Academy of Pediatrics. Recent studies indicate that short courses of doxycycline have negligible risk for tooth staining in young children.[47,48] Skin biopsy of the RMSF eruption may be of diagnostic assistance, as it can demonstrate endothelial damage that progresses into a leukocytoclastic vasculitis, and immunofluorescence may indicate the bacteria in the vessel walls. However, confirmation of a diagnosis is typically achieved during the convalescent stage by documenting a fourfold increase in the IgG on indirect immunofluorescence serologic assay (IFA). IFA has a lower sensitivity during the acute phase of illness, but increases to 94% during the convalescent stage.[49,50] PCR can be performed on skin tissue from biopsy or whole blood but has low sensitivity.[50]

MORBILLIFORM ERUPTION IN THE COVID-19 ERA

Starting in the city of Wuhan, China in December 2019, the novel coronavirus SARS-CoV-2 quickly spread to become a global pandemic, the likes of which had not been seen in more than 100 years. The often-cited "saving grace" of this pandemic has been the low morbidity and mortality documented in children. However, as of the writing of this article, a new inflammatory syndrome termed multisystem inflammatory syndrome in children (MIS-C) is on the increase and an important diagnosis to consider when evaluating a child with new-onset fever and rash. The exact cause of

MIS-C is unknown, but it often occurs 2 to 6 weeks after COVID-19 infection, raising the hypothesis of convalescent immune dysregulation.[51] MIS-C was first described in April 2020 in children within the United Kingdom as an inflammatory syndrome similar to atypical Kawasaki disease (KD) and toxic shock syndrome.[52] One year later, as of April 1, 2021, in the United States, 3185 patients have met the criteria for MIS-C, and 36 patients have died of this disease.[53]

The criteria of MIS-C include age 21 years or younger, fever greater than 38°C, laboratory evidence of inflammation, multisystem organ involvement, and laboratory-confirmed COVID-19 infection (positive RT-PCR testing or antibody test) or epidemiologic link to a person with COVID-19 (**Box 1**).[51] More than half of patients in a targeted surveillance study (n = 186) by Feldstein and colleagues[51] were between 1 and 9 years old with a median age of 8.3 years, although cases in infants and young adults have also been reported. MIS-C disproportionately impacts children of African and Hispanic descent, and obesity has been identified as a risk factor.[54–56] MIS-C commonly presents with fever for 3 to 4 days, gastrointestinal symptoms, mucocutaneous features often seen in KD, and shock. Multisystem organ involvement is a sentinel feature, with 71% of patients having 4 or more systems involved.[51] Gastrointestinal involvement (abdominal pain, vomiting, diarrhea) is the most common organ system (91%–93% of patients) affected. Myocardial dysfunction indicated by either echocardiography or elevated troponin or brain natriuretic peptide is seen in more than 50% of reported cases. Unlike KD, shock is a common feature of MIS-C with 48% of patients requiring vasopressor or vasoactive support throughout their hospital course. Children who present with shock have several distinguishing features, including older age, black race, lack of full criteria for typical or atypical KD, neurologic symptoms, respiratory symptoms, and higher inflammatory markers (specifically, ferritin, C-reactive protein [CRP], and D-dimer).[57]

MIS-C can present with mucocutaneous features that closely resemble those seen in KD. In fact, 40% and 7% of patients with MIS-C meet criteria for typical and atypical KD, respectively.[54] Like KD, conjunctivitis, lip hyperemia/cracking, strawberry tongue, and polymorphic eruptions (urticarial, scarlatiniform, morbilliform) are common features of MIS-C[54] (**Fig. 6**). Periorbital erythema and edema are not characteristically seen in patients with KD, but did occur in 20% of patients with MIS-C, pointing to the possibility of more specific cutaneous findings in this condition.[54] Because of this considerable clinical overlap, distinguishing between KD and MIS-C can be challenging, but, in general, children with MIS-C tend to be older, more likely to have gastrointestinal involvement, myocardial dysfunction, shock, higher inflammatory markers (D-dimer, ferritin, CRP), and tendency toward cytopenia (lymphopenia and thrombocytopenia). Approximately 84% to 90% of patients with MIS-C have positive serologic testing for SARS-CoV-2.[58] The optimal treatment of MIS-C beyond supportive therapy is an area of active investigation.

Box 1
Criteria for diagnosis of multisystem inflammatory syndrome in children

Age <21 y

Fever >38°C

Multisystem organ involvement (≥2 organ systems)

Laboratory evidence of inflammation

COVID-19 PCR-positive/antibody test–positive, OR epidemiologic link to a COVID-19 infected person

Adapted from Feldstein LR, Rose EB, Horwitz SM, Collins JP, Newhams MM, Son MBF, et al. Multisystem Inflammatory Syndrome in US Children and Adolescents. New Engl J Med. 2020;383(4):334 to -46.

MORBILLIFORM ERUPTION WITH A RECENT DRUG HISTORY

A drug history is important to obtain in any patient with a morbilliform eruption. A comprehensive list

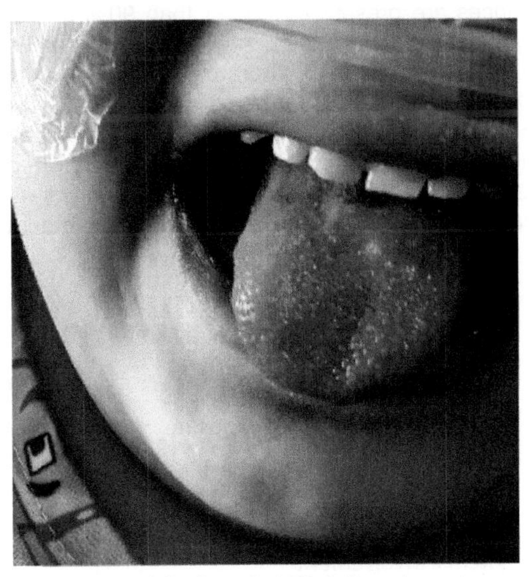

Fig. 6. Mucosal findings in MIS-C. Strawberry tongue and cheilitis in a young child with MIS-C.

of all medications, including over-the-counter medications and supplements, taken with start dates of each is needed to determine probable culprit drugs.

Drug eruptions can be thought of as falling into one of 2 categories: "simple" or "complex." Simple drug eruptions most often occur within 4 days to 2 weeks of starting the medication, and constitutional symptoms or laboratory abnormalities are typically absent. Complex drug eruptions include DRESS, also called drug-induced hypersensitivity disorder, Stevens-Johnson syndrome, and toxic epidermal necrolysis.

Both simple drug eruptions and DRESS syndrome can present with morbilliform rash. The timing and associated systemic symptoms help differentiate these 2 medication reactions. DRESS syndrome usually develops later after exposure to culprit medication, typically 2 to 6 weeks (**Table 3**). The 2 most common features of DRESS are fever and rash. The cutaneous eruption of DRESS is characterized by confluent, erythematous macules and papules.[59] Facial edema serves as an important clue to the diagnosis, seen in around half of patients[60] (**Fig. 7**). Mucous membrane involvement should not be used to rule out the diagnosis. Mucosal involvement (erythema, edema, and erosions) is in fact common (>50%) in both adults and pediatric patients with DRESS, although it rarely progresses to the level of mucosal sloughing seen in Stevens-Johnson syndrome.[59,61] Lymphadenopathy and periorbital edema are common clinical findings in pediatric patients.[61] In most cases, pruritus is common, whereas skin pain is more rare.[60]

In children, hematologic and hepatic disturbances are present in greater than 90% of patients.[61] Although peripheral eosinophilia (>700/μL) is the hallmark laboratory abnormality in DRESS, atypical lymphocytes, thrombocytopenia, thrombocytosis, and anemia can also be documented. Hepatic involvement is reported (elevated AST and ALT) in 80% of children, splenomegaly in 21.5%, and renal involvement in 15.4%.[60] Inflammation of other organ systems, including cardiac, gastrointestinal, musculoskeletal, pulmonary, and the central nervous system, have also been reported.[61] Human herpes virus 6 (HHV-6) reactivation is well documented in DRESS, having been implicated in its pathogenesis, used in clinical criteria, and associated with a more severe disease course in children.[62,63] There are clinical criteria available to aid the clinician in evaluating and diagnosing DRESS.[64]

Antiepileptics are the most common culprit medication (50%), attributed to pediatric DRESS cases, with aromatic antiepileptics accounting for 86.2% of cases owing to this class.[60] Antibiotics are the second most common cause, with vancomycin and trimethoprim-sulfamethoxazole number 1 and 2, respectively.[60] The prompt removal of the offending medication is the gold-standard management of DRESS, and systemic steroids typically tapered over 2 to 6 months are recommended for severe cases.[65,66]

MORBILLIFORM ERUPTIONS IN A BONE MARROW TRANSPLANT PATIENT

A morbilliform eruption in a child with a bone marrow transplant should always be approached with a sense of urgency given the higher risk of acute infection, viral reactivation (cytomegalovirus, Epstein-Barr virus, HHV-6, adenovirus), drug eruption owing to polypharmacy, chemotherapy-induced reactions, and transplant-related rashes, such as acute graft-versus-host disease (GVHD) and engraftment syndrome (ES). GVHD and ES are discussed later, given their uniqueness to this population.

ACUTE GRAFT-VERSUS-HOST DISEASE

Acute GVHD occurs when activated donor immune cells stimulate an inflammatory cascade that leads to host tissue destruction. Acute GVHD is most common in children with

Table 3
Features of simple versus complex morbilliform drug eruptions

	Exanthematous Drug Eruption	DRESS
Timing after medication exposure	4–14 d	2–6 wk
Fever	Uncommon	Common
Facial edema	No	Common
Lymphadenopathy	No	Common
Systemic involvement	No	Yes
Mucosal involvement	Uncommon	Common

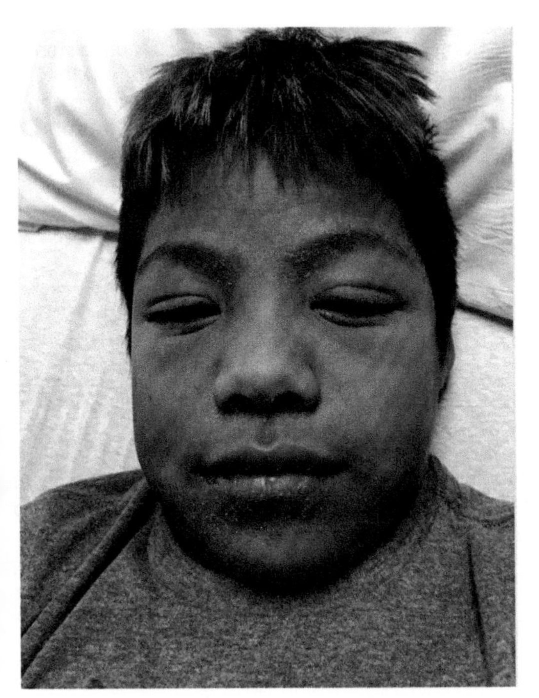

Fig. 7. Erythema, seborrheic scale, and facial edema in a boy with DRESS from ethosuximide.

hematologic malignancies after hematopoietic stem-cell transplantation. According to National Institutes of Health consensus criteria, acute GVHD can be divided into "classic acute GVHD" and "late acute GVHD." "Classic acute GVHD" refers to the development of acute GVHD in the first 100 days following a transplantation. "Late acute GVHD" refers to symptoms of acute GVHD beyond 100 days without features of chronic GVHD. "Late acute GVHD" may be described as "persistent," whereby symptoms of acute GVHD extend beyond 100 days, "recurrent" when a case of classic acute GVHD resolves but then recurs after 100 days, or "de novo" for cases whereby symptoms of acute GVHD only occur for the first time after 100 days.[67] Overall, most cases of acute GVHD coincide with the timing of white blood cell engraftment, occurring around 30 days after transplantation.[68] Organs most commonly affected are the skin, gastrointestinal tract, and the liver, with the skin commonly being first involved.[68] Compared with adults, children have a higher incidence of isolated skin involvement.[52] Mortality in pediatric acute GVHD is highest in recipients of HLA partially matched or mismatched unrelated donor grafts.[68]

Early skin findings of acute GVHD include pink papules on the scalp, pinna of the ears, face, neck, palms, and soles, which may coalesce into larger plaques or become more generalized throughout the body[69] (**Fig. 8**). This morphology

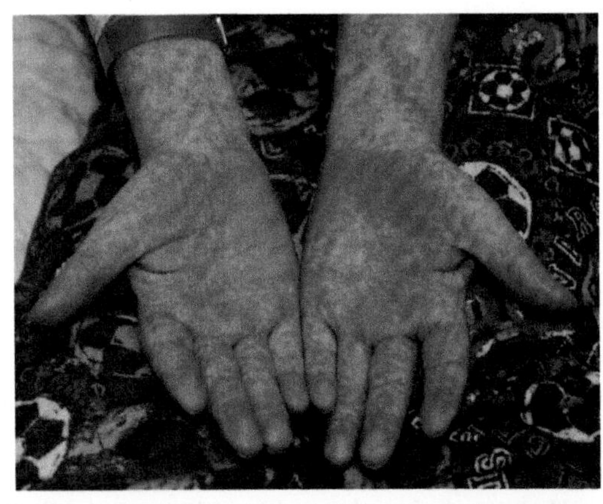

Fig. 8. Acute GVHD. A morbilliform eruption and erythema accentuated on the palms in a child with acute GVHD.

accompanied by diarrhea and/or cholestatic hepatopathy would be the classic presentation for multiorgan involvement of acute GVHD. Histopathological examination of skin biopsies can show changes classic for acute GVHD; however, oftentimes they are more helpful in ruling out alternative diagnoses.[70] One study found that in pediatric patients with concern for acute GVHD, skin biopsies yielded a definitive diagnosis in only 15% of cases, but dermatologic consultation still changed clinical management in 78% of cases.[71]

ENGRAFTMENT SYNDROME

ES can lead to a clinical picture closely resembling acute GVHD. ES is a self-limited, inflammatory syndrome characterized by noninfectious fever, maculopapular exanthem without histologic features of GVHD, and a vascular leak phenomenon leading to weight gain and noncardiogenic pulmonary edema.[72] The pathogenesis of ES is not fully understood but is linked to neutrophil engraftment irrespective of the form of hematologic stem cell transplantation (autologous, allogeneic). Upon engraftment, a proinflammatory cytokine response ensues. ES most commonly occurs 7 to 14 days after transplant, typically 4 days before and 1 day after neutrophil engraftment with autologous or allogeneic stem cells and 7 to 14 days before neutrophil engraftment from umbilical cord stem cell transplantation.

ES cannot be reliably diagnosed based on any histopathologic change or serologic marker. Spitzer[72] has proposed diagnostic criteria for ES (**Box 2**). In the setting of allogeneic transplantation, distinguishing between acute GVHD and ES can be challenging. Onset with days of neutrophil engraftment, responsive to short course of corticosteroids, and pulmonary involvement can be useful clues for diagnosing ES. Whether children

Box 2
Spitzer's criteria for engraftment syndrome

Major criteria

Temperature ≥38.3°C with no identifiable infectious cause

Erythrodermatous rash involving more than 25% of body surface area and not attributable to a medication

Noncardiogenic pulmonary edema, manifested by diffuse pulmonary infiltrates consistent with this diagnosis, and hypoxia

Minor criteria

Hepatic dysfunction with either total bilirubin ≥2 mg/dL or transaminase levels ≥ 2 times normal

Renal insufficiency (serum creatinine of ≥2 times baseline)

Weight gain ≥2.5% of baseline body weight

Transient encephalopathy unexplainable by other causes

Must fulfill all 3 major criteria, or 2 major criteria and 1 or more minor criteria within 96 h of engraftment.

Adapted from Spitzer TR. Engraftment syndrome following hematopoietic stem cell transplantation. Bone Marrow Transplant. 2001 May;27(9):893-8.

with ES are at higher risk for GVHD is controversial and area of active investigation.

SUMMARY

There are many important inflammatory and infectious diagnoses to consider in the hospitalized patient with a morbilliform eruption. The critical goal when evaluating a child with a new-onset morbilliform eruption is to make an accurate diagnosis in a timely manner. Full-body examination and careful history-taking can help to narrow the differential diagnosis and guide the workup.

CLINICS CARE POINTS

- The Koplik spots of measles start 48 hours prior to the onset of the exanthem and last only 12 to 72 hours so maybe absent later in the disease course.
- Doxycycline should be initiated as soon as a diagnosis of Rocky Mountain Spotted fever is being considered independent of the patient's age.
- Compared to Kawasaki disease, Multisystem inflammatory syndrome in children (MIS-C) generally impacts older children who often present with gastrointestinal symptoms, myocardial dysfunction, shock, high inflammatory markes and cytopenias.
- Facial edema is seen in around half of patients with DRESS.
- The eruption of GVHD Often starts on the scalp, ears, face, neck, palms and soles.

DISCLOSURE

V. S. Oza, MD is an editor for Visual Dx regarding Multisystem Inflammatory Syndrome content. Drs S. D. Cipriano and J. S. Haber have nothing to disclose.

REFERENCES

1. Dux A, Lequime S, Patrono LV, et al. Measles virus and rinderpest virus divergence dated to the sixth century BCE. Science 2020;368(6497):1367–70.
2. Cunha BA. Smallpox and measles: historical aspects and clinical differentiation. Infect Dis Clin North Am 2004;18(1):79–100.
3. Cherry JD. Contemporary infectious exanthems. Clin Infect Dis 1993;16(2):199–205.
4. Hinman AR, Orenstein WA, Bloch AB, et al. Impact of measles in the United States. Rev Infect Dis 1983;5(3):439–44.
5. Atkinson WL, Orenstein WA, Krugman S. The resurgence of measles in the United States, 1989-1990. Annu Rev Med 1992;43:451–63.
6. Papania MJ, Wallace GS, Rota PA, et al. Elimination of endemic measles, rubella, and congenital rubella syndrome from the Western hemisphere: the US experience. J Pediatr 2014;168(2):148–55.
7. Roberts L. Why measles deaths are surging - and coronavirus could make it worse. Nature 2020; 580(7804):446–7.
8. Patel M, Lee AD, Redd SB, et al. Increase in measles cases - United States, January 1-April 26, 2019. MMWR Morb Mortal Wkly Rep 2019;68(17): 402–4.
9. Brooks HE, McLendon LA, Daniel CL. The impact of COVID-19 on pediatric vaccination rates in Alabama. Prev Med Rep 2021;22:101320.
10. Yang W. Transmission dynamics of and insights from the 2018-2019 measles outbreak in New York City: a modeling study. Sci Adv 2020;6(22):eaaz4037.
11. Banerjee E, Griffith J, Kenyon C, et al. Containing a measles outbreak in Minnesota, 2017: methods and challenges. Perspect Public Health 2020;140(3): 162–71.

12. Moss WJ. Measles. Lancet 2017;390(10111): 2490–502.
13. Rota PA, Moss WJ, Takeda M, et al. Measles. Nat Rev Dis Primers 2016;2.
14. Roy F, Mendoza L, Hiebert J, et al. Rapid identification of measles virus vaccine genotype by real-time PCR. J Clin Microbiol 2017;55(3):735–43.
15. Bichon A, Aubry C, Benarous L, et al. Case report: ribavirin and vitamin A in a severe case of measles. Medicine (Baltimore) 2017;96(50):e9154.
16. Greenky D, Gillespie S, Levine A, et al. The utility of a travel screen at triage in pediatric emergency medicine. Pediatr Emerg Care 2020; 36(8):384–8.
17. Adams DA, Thomas KR, Jajosky RA, et al. Summary of notifiable infectious diseases and conditions - United States, 2015. MMWR Morb Mortal Wkly Rep 2017;64(53):1–143.
18. Gould E, Pettersson J, Higgs S, et al. Emerging arboviruses: why today? One Health 2017;4:1–13.
19. Wong E, Suarez JA, Naranjo L, et al. Arbovirus rash in the febrile returning traveler as a diagnostic clue. Curr Trop Med Rep 2021;1–8.
20. Young PR. Arboviruses: a family on the move. Adv Exp Med Biol 2018;1062:1–10.
21. Walker WL, Lindsey NP, Lehman JA, et al. Zika virus disease cases - 50 states and the District of Columbia, January 1-July 31, 2016. MMWR Morb Mortal Wkly Rep 2016;65(36):983–6.
22. Centers for Disease C. Zika in the US. 2021. Available at: https://www.cdc.gov/zika/geo/index.html.
23. Duffy MR, Chen TH, Hancock WT, et al. Zika virus outbreak on Yap Island, Federated States of Micronesia. N Engl J Med 2009;360(24):2536–43.
24. Derrington SM, Cellura AP, McDermott LE, et al. Mucocutaneous findings and course in an adult with Zika virus infection. JAMA Dermatol 2016; 152(6):691–3.
25. Ferraris P, Yssel H, Misse D. Zika virus infection: an update. Microbes Infect 2019;21(8–9):353–60.
26. YT-RLCve Mier, Delorey MJ, Sejvar JJ, et al. Guillain-Barre syndrome risk among individuals infected with Zika virus: a multi-country assessment. BMC Med 2018;16(1):67.
27. Burt FJ, Chen WQ, Miner JJ, et al. Chikungunya virus: an update on the biology and pathogenesis of this emerging pathogen. Lancet Infect Dis 2017; 17(4):E107–17.
28. Fischer M, Staples JE. Arboviral Diseases Branch NCfE, Zoonotic Infectious Diseases CDC. Notes from the field: chikungunya virus spreads in the Americas - Caribbean and South America, 2013-2014. MMWR Morb Mortal Wkly Rep 2014;63(22):500–1.
29. Miner JJ, Yeang HXA, Fox JM, et al. Chikungunya viral arthritis in the United States: a mimic of seronegative rheumatoid arthritis. Arthritis Rheum 2015; 67(5):1214–20.
30. Silva LA, Dermody TS. Chikungunya virus: epidemiology, replication, disease mechanisms, and prospective intervention strategies. J Clin Invest 2017; 127(3):737–49.
31. Singal A. Chikungunya and skin: current perspective. Indian Dermatol Online J 2017;8(5):307–9.
32. Friedrich MJ. Asymptomatic people may contribute to Dengue transmission. JAMA 2016;19(3):242.
33. Yacoub S, Wills B. Dengue: an update for clinicians working in non-endemic areas. Clin Med (Lond) 2015;15(1):82–5.
34. Thomas EA, John M, Kanish B. Mucocutaneous manifestations of Dengue fever. Indian J Dermatol 2010;55(1):79–85.
35. Nawas ZY, Tong Y, Kollipara R, et al. Emerging infectious diseases with cutaneous manifestations: viral and bacterial infections. J Am Acad Dermatol 2016;75(1):1–16.
36. Tang KF, Ooi EE. Diagnosis of dengue: an update. Expert Rev Anti Infect Ther 2012;10(8):895–907.
37. Rosenberg R, Lindsey NP, Fischer M, et al. Vital signs: trends in reported vectorborne disease cases - United States and territories, 2004-2016. MMWR Morb Mortal Wkly Rep 2018;67(17): 496–501.
38. Helmick CG, Bernard KW, D'Angelo LJ. Rocky Mountain spotted fever: clinical, laboratory, and epidemiological features of 262 cases. J Infect Dis 1984;150(4):480–8.
39. Dantas-Torres F. Rocky Mountain spotted fever. Lancet Infect Dis 2007;7(11):724–32.
40. Chapman AS, Bakken JS, Folk SM, et al. Diagnosis and management of tickborne rickettsial diseases: Rocky Mountain spotted fever, ehrlichioses, and anaplasmosis–United States: a practical guide for physicians and other health-care and public health professionals. MMWR Recomm Rep 2006;55(RR-4):1–27.
41. Centers for Disease C. Rocky Mountain spotted fever. Available at: https://www.cdc.gov/rmsf/stats/index.html.
42. Hopkins RS, Jajosky RA, Hall PA, et al. Summary of notifiable diseases–United States, 2003. MMWR Morb Mortal Wkly Rep 2005;52(54):1–85.
43. Buckingham SC, Marshall GS, Schutze GE, et al. Clinical and laboratory features, hospital course, and outcome of Rocky Mountain spotted fever in children. J Pediatr 2007;150(2):180–184, 4 e1.
44. Ramos-e-Silva M, Pereira AL. Life-threatening eruptions due to infectious agents. Clin Dermatol 2005; 23(2):148–56.
45. Kirkland KB, Wilkinson WE, Sexton DJ. Therapeutic delay and mortality in cases of Rocky Mountain spotted fever. Clin Infect Dis 1995;20(5):1118–21.
46. Tull R, Ahn C, Daniel A, et al. Retrospective study of Rocky Mountain spotted fever in children. Pediatr Dermatol 2017;34(2):119–23.

47. Lochary ME, Lockhart PB, Williams WT Jr. Doxycycline and staining of permanent teeth. Pediatr Infect Dis J 1998;17(5):429–31.
48. Todd SR, Dahlgren FS, Traeger MS, et al. No visible dental staining in children treated with doxycycline for suspected Rocky Mountain spotted fever. J Pediatr 2015;166(5):1246–51.
49. Kaplan JE, Schonberger LB. The sensitivity of various serologic tests in the diagnosis of Rocky Mountain spotted fever. Am J Trop Med Hyg 1986;35(4):840–4.
50. Biggs HM, Behravesh CB, Bradley KK, et al. Diagnosis and management of tickborne rickettsial diseases: Rocky Mountain spotted fever and other spotted fever group rickettsioses, ehrlichioses, and anaplasmosis - United States. MMWR Recomm Rep 2016;65(2):1–44.
51. Feldstein LR, Rose EB, Horwitz SM, et al. Multisystem inflammatory syndrome in US children and adolescents. N Engl J Med 2020;383(4):334–46.
52. Riphagen S, Gomez X, Gonzalez-Martinez C, et al. Hyperinflammatory shock in children during COVID-19 pandemic. Lancet 2020;395(10237):1607–8.
53. Centers for Disease C. Health Department-reported cases of multisystem inflammatory syndrome in children (MIS-C) in the United States. 2021. Available at: https://www.cdc.gov/mis-c/cases/index.html.
54. Young TK, Shaw KS, Shah JK, et al. Mucocutaneous manifestations of multisystem inflammatory syndrome in children during the COVID-19 pandemic. JAMA Dermatol 2021;157(2):207–12.
55. Abrams JY, Oster ME, Godfred-Cato SE, et al. Factors linked to severe outcomes in multisystem inflammatory syndrome in children (MIS-C) in the USA: a retrospective surveillance study. Lancet Child Adolesc Health 2021;5(5):323–31.
56. Godfred-Cato S, Bryant B, Leung J, et al. COVID-19-associated multisystem inflammatory syndrome in children - United States, March-July 2020. MMWR Morb Mortal Wkly Rep 2020;69(32):1074–80.
57. Bautista-Rodriguez C, Sanchez-de-Toledo J, Clark BC, et al. Multisystem inflammatory syndrome in children: an international survey. Pediatrics 2021;147(2).
58. Ahmed M, Advani S, Moreira A, et al. Multisystem inflammatory syndrome in children: a systematic review. EClinicalMedicine 2020;26:100527.
59. Kardaun SH, Sekula P, Valeyrie-Allanore L, et al. Drug reaction with eosinophilia and systemic symptoms (DRESS): an original multisystem adverse drug reaction. Results from the prospective RegiSCAR study. Br J Dermatol 2013;169(5):1071–80.
60. Metterle L, Hatch L, Seminario-Vidal L. Pediatric drug reaction with eosinophilia and systemic symptoms: a systematic review of the literature. Pediatr Dermatol 2020;37(1):124–9.
61. Newell BD, Moinfar M, Mancini AJ, et al. Retrospective analysis of 32 pediatric patients with anticonvulsant hypersensitivity syndrome (ACHSS). Pediatr Dermatol 2009;26(5):536–46.
62. Ahluwalia J, Abuabara K, Perman MJ, et al. Human herpesvirus 6 involvement in paediatric drug hypersensitivity syndrome. Br J Dermatol 2015;172(4):1090–5.
63. Tohyama M, Hashimoto K, Yasukawa M, et al. Association of human herpesvirus 6 reactivation with the flaring and severity of drug-induced hypersensitivity syndrome. Br J Dermatol 2007;157(5):934–40.
64. Husain Z, Reddy BY, Schwartz RA. DRESS syndrome: part I. Clinical perspectives. J Am Acad Dermatol 2013;68(5):693 e1–14.
65. Roujeau JC, Haddad C, Paulmann M, et al. Management of nonimmediate hypersensitivity reactions to drugs. Immunol Allergy Clin N Am 2014;34(3):473–487, vii.
66. Husain Z, Reddy BY, Schwartz RA. DRESS syndrome: part II. Management and therapeutics. J Am Acad Dermatol 2013;68(5). 709 e1-9.
67. Jagasia MH, Greinix HT, Arora M, et al. National Institutes of Health Consensus Development Project on Criteria for Clinical Trials in Chronic Graft-versus-Host Disease: I. The 2014 Diagnosis and Staging Working Group report. Biol Blood Marrow Transplant 2015;21(3):389–401.e1.
68. MacMillan ML, Holtan SG, Rashidi A, et al. Pediatric acute GVHD: clinical phenotype and response to upfront steroids. Bone Marrow Transplant 2020;55(1):165–71.
69. Johnson ML, Farmer ER. Graft-versus-host reactions in dermatology. J Am Acad Dermatol 1998;38(3):369–92.
70. Paun O, Phillips T, Fu P, et al. Cutaneous complications in hematopoietic cell transplant recipients: impact of biopsy on patient management. Biol Blood Marrow Transplant 2013;19(8):1204–9.
71. Haimes H, Morley KW, Song H, et al. Impact of skin biopsy on the management of acute graft-versus-host disease in a pediatric population. Pediatr Dermatol 2019;36(4):455–9.
72. Spitzer TR. Engraftment syndrome: double-edged sword of hematopoietic cell transplants. Bone Marrow Transplant 2015;50(4):469–75.

Supportive Oncodermatology in Pediatric Patients

Danny W. Linggonegoro, BS[a,b], Hannah Song, MD[a,b], Jennifer T. Huang, MD[a,b,*]

KEYWORDS

• Oncodermatology • Targeted therapy • Pediatric dermatology • Cutaneous reaction • Management

KEY POINTS

- Targeted cancer therapies block specific molecular pathways involved in the growth, progression, and spread of cancer.
- Pediatric dermatology literature is emerging on the specific types and prevalence of cutaneous reactions to targeted therapies that hone in on membrane-bound receptors (eg, BCR-ABL, EGFR, or SMO inhibitors), intracellular signaling targets (eg, BRAF, MEK, mTOR), and antiangiogenesis agents (eg, VEGF), as well as targeted immunotherapies.
- Information about the timing, severity, and treatment algorithm for these cutaneous reactions is most well described for BRAF, MEK, and EGFR inhibitors.
- Further research on the most common cutaneous reactions of targeted therapy in children, potential treatments, and prevention is crucial to better serve the needs of this population.

INTRODUCTION

Cancer is an important cause of morbidity and mortality in children.[1] Targeted therapies have been developed to hone in on specific molecular pathways involved in the growth, progression, and spread of cancer. Although targeted therapies have become a focus of current anticancer drug development and are being increasingly used in pediatric populations, different cutaneous side effects have emerged with use of these therapies. Some targeted therapies result in dermatologic adverse events in nearly all treated children. Common reactions include xerosis, follicular and/or eczematous reactions, and hand-foot skin reactions. However, a subset of patients will experience adverse cutaneous effects that have the potential to lead to treatment cessation. In the authors' clinical experience, most children can be treated with topical and/or oral therapies without treatment breaks or cessation. Only rarely will children experience severe drug hypersensitivity reactions with internal organ involvement or Stevens-Johnson syndrome-like reactions requiring permanent drug cessation. Understanding the most common cutaneous reactions of targeted therapy in children and their treatments is crucial to better serve the needs of this population. In this article, the authors review common side effects of select targeted therapies and offer treatment options.

DISCUSSION

Types of Targeted Therapies, Prevalence of Cutaneous Reactions, Management

Targeted therapies are a type of cancer treatment that acts on membrane-bound receptors or intracellular signals to interfere with specific proteins that help tumors proliferate without regulation and resist apoptosis (**Fig. 1**).[3] The focus of this article is reactions to monotherapy with targeted therapeutics; however, combination therapy of different agents will also be discussed.

[a] Boston Children's Hospital, Dermatology Program, 300 Longwood Avenue, Fegan 6, Boston, MA 02115, USA;
[b] Harvard Medical School, 25 Shattuck St, Boston, MA 02115, USA
* Corresponding author. 300 Longwood Avenue, Fegan 6, Boston, MA 02115.
E-mail address: Jennifer.Huang@childrens.harvard.edu

Dermatol Clin 40 (2022) 203–214
https://doi.org/10.1016/j.det.2021.12.007
0733-8635/22/© 2021 Elsevier Inc. All rights reserved.

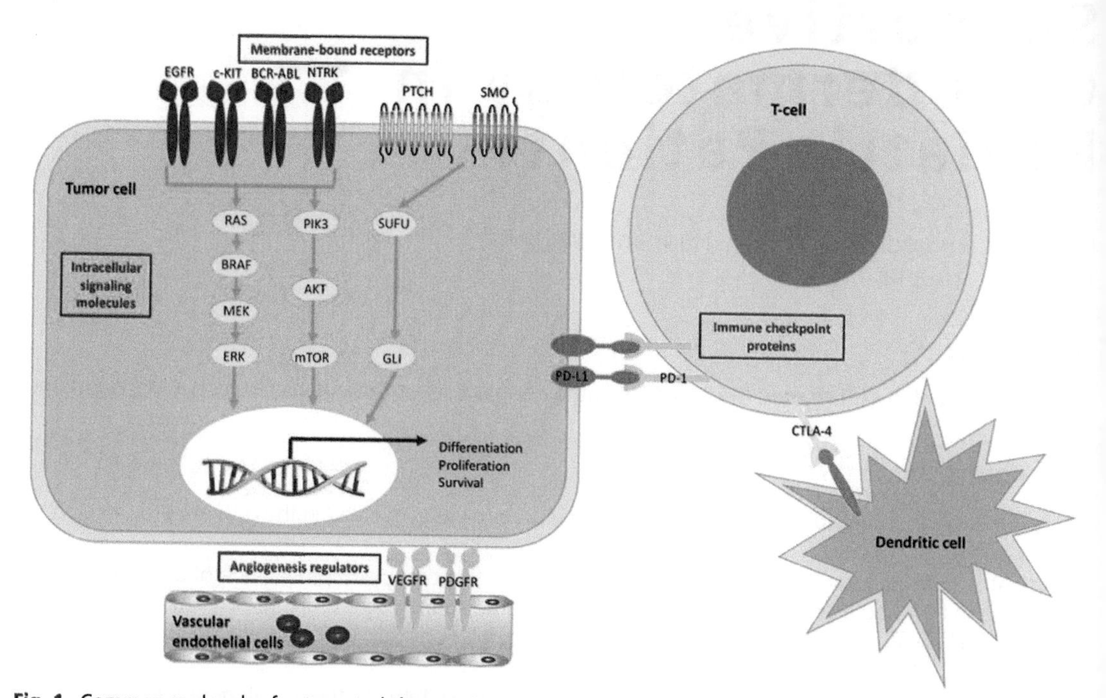

Fig. 1. Common molecules for targeted therapy in cancer. Therapies target membrane-bound receptors, intracellular signaling molecules, angiogenesis mediators, and immune checkpoint proteins to inhibit various steps of oncogenesis. From Carlberg, and colleagues; with permission from John Wiley & Sons.[2]

Classes of medications and brief mechanisms of action are reviewed. Each section includes incidence of cutaneous findings. Medication-specific treatment options are discussed in this section if any are available (**Table 1**). There are limited randomized clinical trials evaluating the effectiveness of management of cutaneous reactions in pediatric patients. Only reactions observed in pediatric patients are included. Dose reductions or switching to a different medication in the same class may be helpful for all these cutaneous reactions. Severe blistering skin reactions or skin reactions with internal organ involvement should prompt drug cessation. Dermatologists should work closely with oncologists to manage these complex patients.

Membrane-Bound Receptors or Intracellular Signaling Molecules

Most targeted therapies are monoclonal antibodies or small-molecule drugs. Monoclonal antibodies target specific proteins on the surface of cancerous cells. Small-molecule drugs target specific substances inside the cell.

Membrane-bound receptors

Tyrosine kinase receptors: BCR-ABL inhibitors BCR-ABL inhibitors used in children include imatinib, dasatinib, and nilotinib. Translocation between the ABL tyrosine kinase gene on chromosome 9 and BCR gene on chromosome 22 leads to an oncogenic BCR-ABL1 fusion gene in hematopoietic stem cells. This fusion gene encodes a BCR-ABL protein kinase with constitutive tyrosine kinase activity leading to proliferative and antiapoptotic signaling responsible for hematologic malignancies.[4]

A maculopapular rash has been reported in 1.7% to 45.5% of pediatric patients.[5] Grade 1 to 2 periorbital edema has been reported in 25% of pediatric patients receiving imatinib.[6] Imatinib has a high degree of specificity for the platelet-derived growth factor receptor tyrosine kinase family, which is thought to regulate tissue fluid properties and is highly expressed in the dermal dendrocytes of periorbital tissue.[7] Rare cutaneous reactions include mucositis (6%), pruritus (2.3%), and madarosis (3%) in pediatric patients on BCR-ABL inhibitors.[5,8] Hypopigmentation has been reported in 1 case of a child with chronic myeloid leukemia being treated with imatinib.[9] The keratosis pilaris-like eruption associated with BCR-ABL has the characteristic perifollicular appearance, is generalized, and is variably associated with pruritus. In contrast, typical keratosis pilaris has a predilection for the lateral upper arms and legs and is usually asymptomatic. Pseudoporphyria has also been described in a few cases of children and adults receiving imatinib.[10] The onset of pseudoporphyria, occurring at months to years after imatinib initiation, appears to be significantly delayed compared with the other more commonly reported cutaneous reactions.[10] Dose reduction or cessation of imatinib resulted in complete resolution of the pseudoporphyria.[10]

Table 1
Summary of dermatologic adverse events of targeted therapies and proposed management; management depends on the extent, severity, and underlying cause of the cutaneous reaction

Cutaneous Toxicities	Agents	Proposed Management
Maculopapular, acneiform, papulopustular rash	EGFR inhibitors[a] BCR-ABL inhibitors[a] SMO inhibitors BRAF inhibitors MEK inhibitors[a] mTOR inhibitors[a] AKT inhibitors VEGF receptor tyrosine kinase inhibitors CTLA-4 inhibitors	• Preemptive use of emollients, sunscreen, oral antibiotics, and topical steroids may be helpful Mild: • Topical steroids • Topical antimicrobial wash (benzoyl peroxide) • Dilute bleach baths • Emollients • Photoprotection Moderate: • Oral antibiotics • Culture-driven antibiotics if secondary infection Severe: • Oral isotretinoin
Subcutaneous edema (periorbital, peripheral)	BCR-ABL inhibitors BRAF inhibitors mTOR inhibitors	• Limit salt intake • Compression stockings • Topical steroids • Diuretics • Topical phenylephrine • Blepharoplasty for severe cases of periorbital edema
Mucosal changes (mucositis, angular cheilitis)	BCR-ABL inhibitors MEK inhibitors AKT inhibitors mTOR	• Antiseptic mouthwash without alcohol • Topical analgesics • Topical steroids • Liquid, soft, or normal diet as tolerated
Pruritus	BCR-ABL inhibitors EGFR inhibitors AKT inhibitors VEGF receptor tyrosine kinase inhibitors CTLA-4 inhibitors	• Emollients • Topical steroids • Gentle skin care (short, warm showers; nonfragrance soaps; nonfragrance detergents) • Oral antihistamines
Madarosis	BCR-ABL inhibitors SMO inhibitors	• Usually reversible once responsible agent is discontinued • Topical minoxidil
Hypopigmentation	BCR-ABL inhibitors SMO inhibitors	• Usually reversible once responsible agent is discontinued
Keratosis pilaris-like eruption	BCR-ABL inhibitors BRAF inhibitors	• Topical emollients • Topical keratolytics • Isotretinoin
Pseudoporphyria	BCR-ABL inhibitors	• Photoprotection • Dose reduction or change targeted therapy
Xerosis	EGFR inhibitors BRAF inhibitors MEK inhibitors mTOR inhibitors AKT inhibitors VEGF receptor tyrosine kinase inhibitors CTLA-4 inhibitors	• Emollients • Gentle skin care (short, warm showers; nonfragrance soaps; nonfragrance detergents)

(*continued on next page*)

Table 1
(*continued*)

Cutaneous Toxicities	Agents	Proposed Management
Trichomegaly	EGFR inhibitors	• Regular trimming and epilation to prevent obscuring vision, corneal erosions, irritation, and infection
Hypertrichosis	EGFR inhibitors	• Regular trimming
Alopecia	EGFR inhibitors SMO inhibitors BRAF inhibitors MEK inhibitors VEGF receptor tyrosine kinase inhibitors	• Topical minoxidil • Usually reversible once responsible agent is discontinued
Hyperhidrosis	SMO inhibitors CTLA-4 inhibitors	• Antiperspirants, topical anticholinergics • Oral anticholinergics
Photosensitivity	BRAF inhibitors MEK inhibitors	• Photoprotection
Hand-foot skin reaction	BRAF inhibitors mTOR inhibitors VEGF receptor tyrosine kinase inhibitors	• Topical steroids • Topical keratolytics • Emollients • Topical analgesics • Avoid friction of pressure points (thick socks and comfortable shoes)
Hair changes (changes in color or texture)	BRAF inhibitors MEK inhibitors VEGF receptor tyrosine kinase inhibitors	• Usually reversible once responsible agent is discontinued
Eruptive nevi	BRAF inhibitors MEK inhibitors	• Photoprotection • Baseline and routine skin examinations
Neutrophilic panniculitis	BRAF inhibitors	• Oral analgesics • Compression garments • Oral steroids • Injected steroids • Elevation of affected area
Hyperpigmentation	BRAF inhibitors	• Usually reversible once responsible agent is discontinued • Photoprotection
Delayed wound healing	BRAF inhibitors VEGF inhibitors	• Hold agent for 1 mo after surgery or until wound has healed
Paronychia	MEK inhibitors EGFR inhibitors mTOR inhibitors	• Gentle nail care (regular trimming once a week for fingernails and once a month for toenails; trim nails after showering; avoid trauma) • Dilute bleach soaks • Silver nitrate • Topical steroids • Culture driven topical or oral antibiotics

[a] Most common medications with the associated dermatologic adverse reaction.

Tyrosine kinase receptors: neurotrophic receptor tyrosine kinase inhibitors Neurotrophic receptor tyrosine kinase (NTRK) inhibitors in children include entrectinib and larotrectinib. NTRK oncogenic fusions promote tumorigenesis via constitutive ligand-free activation of intracellular pathways that control cell-cycle progression, proliferation, apoptosis, and survival.[11,12] NTRK fusions are seen more frequently in pediatric tumors than in adult tumors.[13] These pediatric tumors include infantile fibrosarcoma, cellular congenital mesoblastic nephroma, and papillary thyroid cancer.[13] Ongoing clinical trials are evaluating the optimal use of these drugs in children with NTRK fusions.[14] No cutaneous adverse effects have yet been reported with use of this targeted therapy.

Tyrosine kinase receptors: EGFR inhibitors Epidermal growth factor receptor (EGFR) inhibitors in children include erlotinib, cetuximab, gefitinib, and lapatinib. Acneiform rash is the most common type of skin toxicity reported in pediatric trials, with a prevalence of up to 67%.[15,16] Other common side effects include xerosis (48%), erythema (45%), pruritus (17%–21%), and trichomegaly (17%).[16] Clinical details regarding "erythema" were not available. Other rarer adverse reactions include hypertrichosis, alopecia, and cutaneous infection.[16] A study in pediatric patients receiving rapamycin and erlotinib reported 10% incidence of paronychia.[17] Time of onset of these cutaneous reactions in the pediatric population has not been described, but occurs within the first few weeks of treatment in adults.[18]

Practice guidelines for prevention and treatment of EGFR-inhibitor–associated dermatologic toxicities derive from approaches in adults (**Table 2**). Preemptive management of skin toxicity with emollients, sunscreen, oral doxycycline, and topical steroids showed a 50% decrease in the incidence of grade greater than 2 skin toxicities compared with the incidence in those who had reactive management of the cutaneous reactions.[19–21]

G-protein-coupled receptor: smoothened inhibitors Aberrant Hedgehog signaling has been implicated in carcinogenesis with a markedly increased risk of advanced basal cell carcinoma and medulloblastoma.[22,23] Although smoothened (SMO) inhibitors are not currently approved for pediatric patients, there are 2 clinical trials evaluating vismodegib and sonidegib for pediatric cancer.[24] Although sonidegib was well tolerated, premature growth plate changes were observed in prepubertal pediatric patients, which has limited their use.[24]

Cutaneous effects reported in a phase I and II clinical trial in children receiving sonidegib include alopecia (8.3%), madarosis (6.7%), and nail disorder (3.3%). Preliminary data in an ongoing trial in children receiving vismodegib have shown other cutaneous adverse effects, including hyperhidrosis, purpura, acneiform rash, and skin hypopigmentation.[25]

Intracellular signaling targets

Mitogen activated protein kinase pathway: BRAF inhibitors BRAF inhibitors include vemurafenib and dabrafenib. The estimated prevalence of cutaneous reaction in patients receiving BRAF inhibitors is nearly 100% in children, and there are usually multiple reactions.[26,27] Time to onset of cutaneous reactions in children is not clear, but occurs within days to weeks in adults after initiation of BRAF inhibitors.[28] The most common cutaneous side effects of these agents include follicular eruptions, which impact 55% to 100% of patients receiving BRAF inhibitors. The follicular eruptions can present with keratosis pilaris-like reactions or comedonal eruptions and are typically distributed on the extremities and scalp.[26,27] Pruritic xerotic/eczematous dermatitis (36%–50%), photosensitivity (36%), hand-foot skin reactions (**Fig. 2**) with hyperkeratosis of pressure points of the palms and soles (36%–83%), and hair changes (changes in color or texture and alopecia; 30%) are other common cutaneous reactions. Inflammatory papules and pustules occurred in 18% of patients and were less common in children younger than 8 years (5%).[4,5] Other rarer reactions that have been reported include the following: eruptive nevi (23%) (**Fig. 3**), neutrophilic panniculitis (16%), periorbital edema, hyperpigmentation, delayed wound healing, erythema multiforme-like reaction, and severe photosensitivity reaction.[7]

Mitogen activated protein kinase pathway: MEK inhibitors MEK inhibitors include trametinib, cobimetinib, binimetinib, and selumetinib. In addition to cancer therapy, selumetinib has been approved by the Food and Drug Administration (FDA) for treatment of plexiform neurofibromas associated with neurofibromatosis-1. The estimated prevalence of cutaneous reactions in pediatric patients on an MEK inhibitor is 100%. Common reactions include acneiform eruptions (67%–87%) (**Figs. 4** and **5**), xerosis (58%–72.7%), and paronychia (36%–51%) (**Fig. 6**).[26,27] Other less common reactions include hair changes, including alopecia, curly hair texture, and hair lightening (18%–23.3%), seborrheic dermatitis (26%), folliculitis (19%), and angular cheilitis (7%–27.3%). Other rarer reactions (<10% prevalence) include photosensitivity, eruptive nevi, oral mucositis, nail changes, excess facial hair, psoriasiform eruption, and drug rash with eosinophilia and systemic symptoms-like reaction.

PI3K/AKT/mTOR pathway: phosphatidylinositol-4,5-bisphosphate 3-kinase inhibitors PI3K activates a signaling cascade that controls cellular proliferation, survival, and motility. PTEN is one of the more common inactivated tumor suppressor genes. Mutations in PTEN lead to lack of control of PIP3 levels and constitutive activation of

Table 2
Epidermal growth factor receptor inhibitor associated acneiform rash treatment algorithm with grading based on the National Cancer Institute Common Terminology for Adverse Events, version 4.0

Grade of Acneiform Rash	Approach to Treatment
Grade 1: Papules and/or pustules covering <10% of the body surface area (BSA) with or without symptoms of pruritus or tenderness	• Emollients • Photo-protection • Low-potency topical steroids twice a day • Topical antibiotics (clindamycin gel 1%, erythromycin gel/cream 3%; metronidazole cream/gel 0.75%–1%) twice a day for 4 wk • If not improved, treat it as grade 2 rash
Grade 2: Papules and/or pustules covering 10%–30% of the BSA with or without symptoms of pruritus or tenderness; with psychosocial impact	• Oral antibiotics (doxycycline 200 mg or minocycline 200 mg daily) for 4–6 wk • If not improved, treat it as grade 3 rash
Grade ≥3: Papules and/or pustules covering >30% of the BSA with or without symptoms of pruritus or tenderness; limiting self-care activities of daily living	• Low-dose isotretinoin (20–30 mg daily) for 2 mo • If rash interferes with self-care activities, adjusting the dose of EGFR inhibitor until rash improves may be considered

Data from Lupu I, Voiculescu V, Bacalbasa N, Prie B, Cojocaru I, Giurcaneanu C. Cutaneous adverse reactions specific to epidermal growth factor receptor inhibitors. J Med Life. 2015;8(Spec Issue):57-61.

PI3K signaling.[29] Currently, there are clinical trials in pediatric patients with osteosarcoma or Ewing sarcoma evaluating PI3K inhibitors BAY80-6946 and LY3023414; however, no cutaneous reactions have been reported.[30–32]

PI3K/AKT/mTOR pathway: AKT inhibitors AKT is activated downstream of PI3K, which transmits signals from cytokines, growth factors, and oncoproteins to multiple targets. AKT inhibitors include miransertib, perifosine, miltefosine, and MK2206. AKT inhibitors have been studied in children with proteus syndrome, ovarian carcinoma, and visceral leishmaniasis. Although there are no robust data describing cutaneous reactions of AKT inhibitors, mucositis, xerosis, pruritus, and maculopapular rash have been observed in a small sample of children receiving AKT inhibitors.[33,34]

PI3K/AKT/mTOR pathway: mechanistic target of rapamycin inhibitors Mechanistic target of rapamycin (mTOR) is activated further downstream of AKT. The mTOR inhibitors include everolimus, sirolimus, temsirolimus, and ridaforolimus. The most common cutaneous reaction in children taking mTOR inhibitors is mucositis, occurring in 83% of patients in a phase I study with 60% having a grade 3 adverse effect.[35] Xerosis occurred in 80% of pediatric patients. Other cutaneous side effects of mTOR inhibitors in children include follicular rash, nail changes, paronychia, hand-foot skin reaction, and peripheral edema.[27,36–40] A proposed treatment algorithm for cutaneous reactions for BRAF, MEK, and mTOR inhibitors includes baseline gentle skin care and sun protection (**Fig. 7**).

Antiangiogenesis

Angiogenesis is a critical step in tumor growth and metastasis. Before a tumor can grow more than 1 to 2 mm, its cells require blood vessels for nutrients and oxygen.[41,42] Antiangiogenic agents target protein expression, receptors, and ligands in the vascular endothelial growth factor (VEGF) signaling pathway.

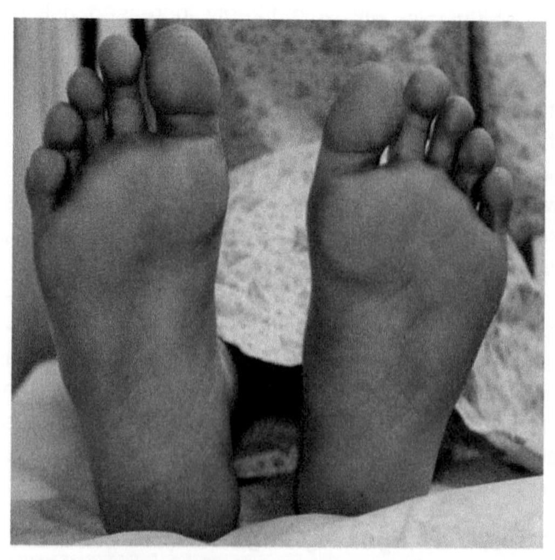

Fig. 2. Hand-foot skin reaction in a patient on a BRAF inhibitor.

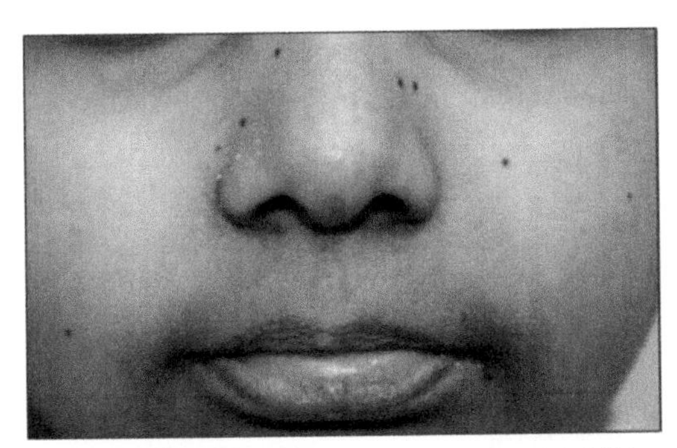

Fig. 3. Eruptive nevi in a patient on a BRAF inhibitor.

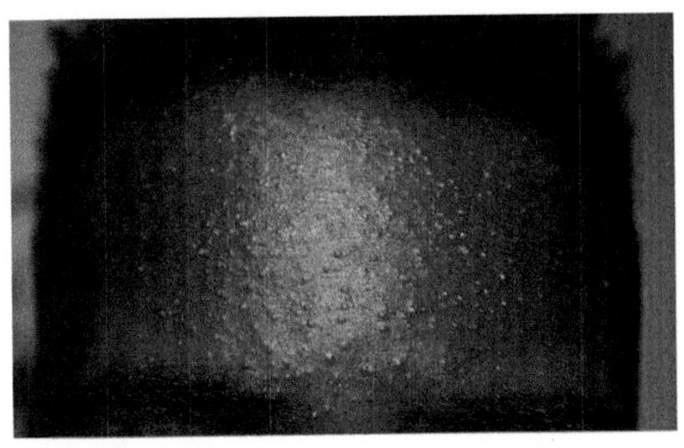

Fig. 5. Mild acneiform rash on the forehead in a patient receiving trametinib.

Vascular endothelial growth factor and vascular endothelial growth factor receptor inhibitors VEGF is a key mediator of vascular development in physiologic growth and embryogenesis; it also plays an important role in pathologic angiogenesis. VEGF is expressed ubiquitously in nearly all human cancers to date. Currently, it is the best-characterized proangiogenic cytokine.[41] Higher levels of VEGF have been associated with increased tumor vascularity, as well as rapid tumor growth, invasion, and metastasis. Blocking the VEGF pathway has thus been an important area of cancer drug development. Bevacizumab was the first anti-VEGF monoclonal antibody approved by the FDA and is one of the best-characterized VEGF inhibitors.

For patients taking bevacizumab after tumor resection, delayed wound healing was one of the more commonly reported adverse effects.[43] Surgical wound dehiscence and enterocutaneous fistula have also been reported.[44,45] Dehiscence of high-dose corticosteroid-induced striae at nonsurgical sites has been reported in 2 children receiving bevacizumab.[46,47] Some experts report that bevacizumab therapy should be delayed until complete surgical site healing or 4 weeks after surgery to avoid these complications.

Multikinase inhibitors: vascular endothelial growth factor receptor tyrosine kinase inhibitors VEGF receptor tyrosine kinase inhibitors currently being investigated for treatment of pediatric hematologic malignancy and solid tumors include sorafenib, sunitinib, and pazopanib.[48(p2)] Preliminary data reveal dose-limiting toxicities, including hand-foot skin reaction and maculopapular rash.[49] When sorafenib was administered concurrently with clofarabine and cytarabine, up to 67% of patients developed grade 2 hand-foot skin reaction or higher.[50] Increased pressure and friction, such as in the setting of wearing hard orthotics, may increase the risk of developing hand-foot skin reaction.[51] Up to 83% of patients on sorafenib monotherapy developed a maculopapular rash, and 50% developed xerosis.[52] Other cutaneous reactions associated with sorafenib monotherapy include lip discoloration, alopecia, hair color changes, and pruritus.[52–54] Hair color changes, most commonly in the form of pigmentary dilution, was the most common cutaneous

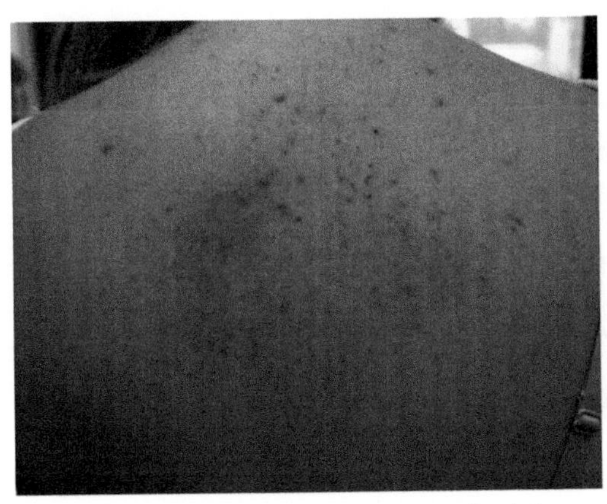

Fig. 4. Mild acneiform rash on the upper back in a patient receiving trametinib.

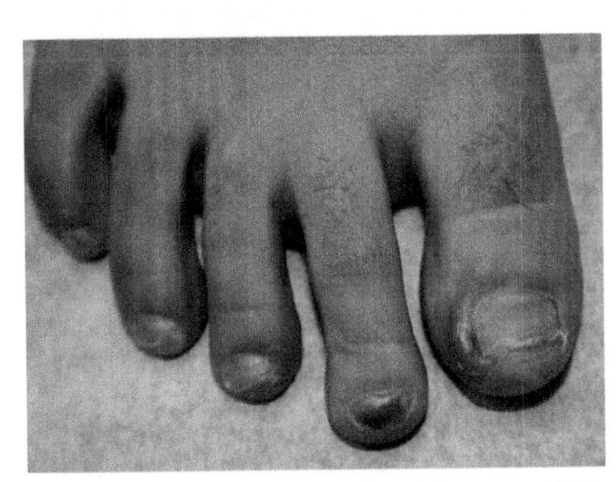

Fig. 6. Paronychia in a patient receiving trametinib.

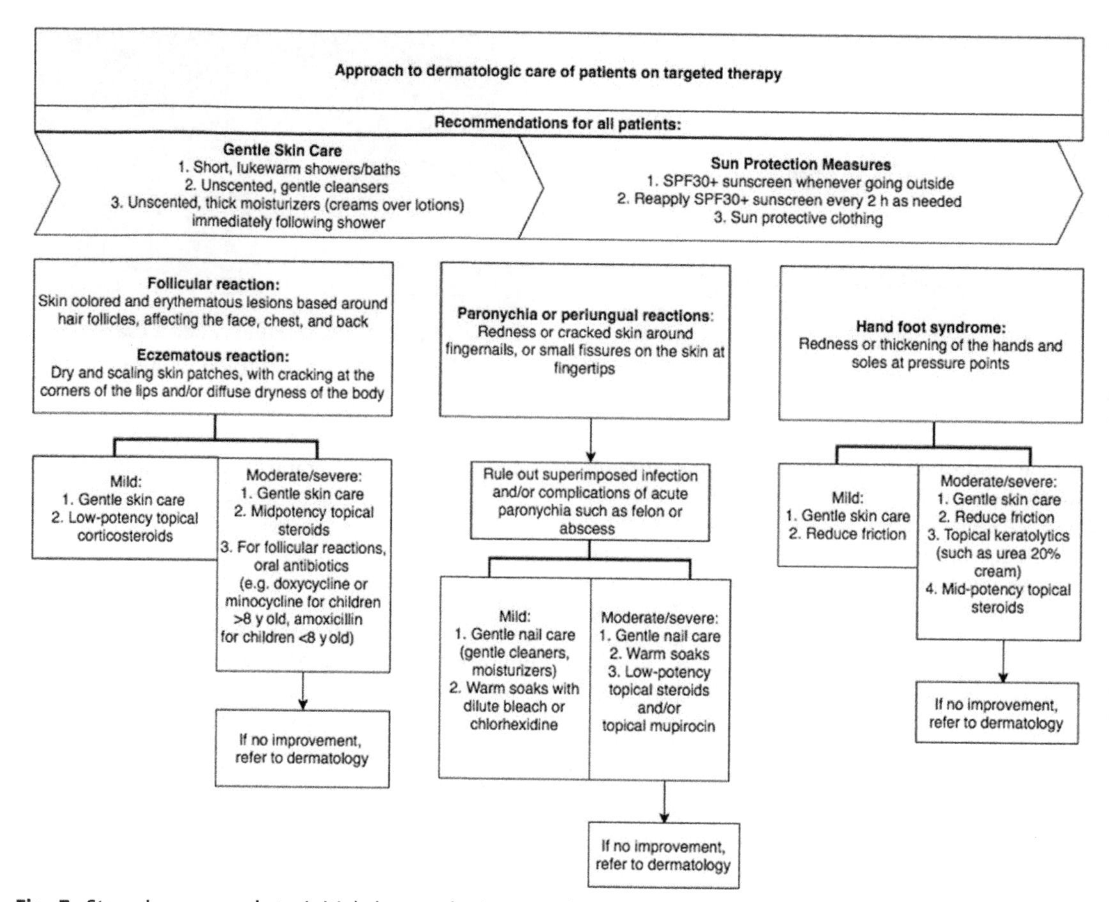

Fig. 7. Stepwise approach to initial dermatologic care of pediatric patients on BRAF, MEK or mTOR inhibitor monotherapy. (From Song H, Zhong CS, Kieran MW, Chi SN, Wright KD, Huang JT. Cutaneous reactions to targeted therapies in children with CNS tumors: A cross-sectional study. Pediatr Blood Cancer. 2019;66(6):e27682.)

adverse effect associated in pediatric patients receiving pazopanib (**Fig. 8**).[55] Other less common cutaneous effects include rash, urticaria, hand-foot skin reaction, xerosis, and generalized hypopigmentation. Notably, the incidence of cutaneous reactions with sorafenib is higher compared with pazopanib and sunitinib.[56] Patients receiving sorafenib also had the highest incidence of grade $\geq$3 rash compared with other VEGF receptor tyrosine kinase inhibitors.[56]

A clinical trial for treatment of sorafenib-induced hand-foot skin reaction with urea cream is currently underway.[57]

Targeted immunotherapy

The immune system is able to detect and defend against abnormal cells, including cancerous cells. Tumor-infiltrating lymphocytes or TILs are found in and around tumors, and the presence of TILs are a positive prognostic indicator for oncology patients. Some cancerous cells can evade the immune system through mechanisms like genetic mutations to make themselves less detectable by immune cells. Targeted immunotherapy has been developed to upregulate the anticancer response. This section discusses the more recently developed dermatologic adverse effects of immune checkpoint

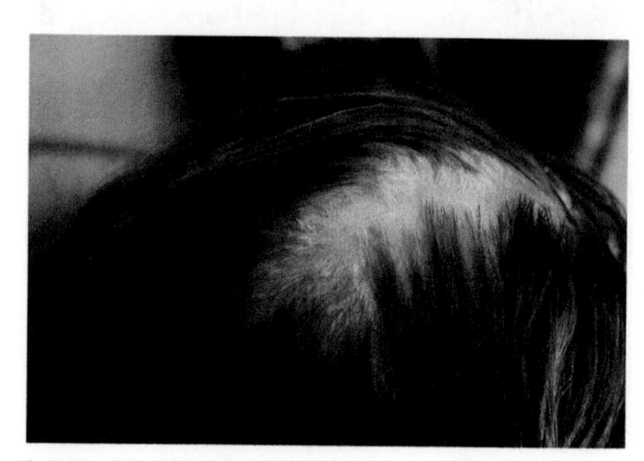

Fig. 8. Pigmentary dilution in a patient receiving pazopanib.

inhibitors, including inhibitors of cytotoxic T-lymphocyte-associated protein 4 (CTLA-4), programmed death protein 1 (PD-1), and programmed death ligand 1 (PD-L1). The checkpoint proteins CTLA-4 and PD-1 are located on T cells and downregulate autoimmune responses. PD-L1 is a protein on the surface of cancer cells in addition to some normal cells. PD-1 on T cells binds to its partner protein PD-L1 on normal and/or cancer cells and thereby dampens the T-cell response. Checkpoint inhibitors work by blocking these checkpoint proteins from binding with their partner proteins, which prevents T cells from being downregulated and augments the immune response.

Checkpoint inhibitors: cytotoxic T-lymphocyte-associated protein 4 inhibitors Ipilimumab is a CTLA-4 inhibitor approved for use in pediatric patients 12 years of age or older.[58] A phase II trial of children between ages 12 and 18 years with stage III to IV malignant melanoma showed more cutaneous reactions in children taking 10 mg/kg versus children taking 3 mg/kg. These patients developed acne, xerosis, hyperhidrosis, pruritus, and rash.[59] Details describing the morphology of the rash were not available. Another phase II trial reported no grade 3 or 4 dermatologic adverse effects for children receiving treatment with ipilimumab.[60]

Checkpoint inhibitors: programmed death protein-1 and programmed death ligand-1 inhibitors PD-L1 inhibitors approved in pediatric populations include atezolizumab, avelumab, and durvalumab. In patients receiving nivolumab, several dermatologic adverse events were reported: maculopapular rash (11%), mucositis (1%), and Stevens-Johnson syndrome (1%).[61] In pediatric patients receiving pembrolizumab, dermatologic adverse events included rash (8%), pruritus (2%), and photosensitivity reaction (<1%).[62] In another retrospective cohort study with pediatric patients receiving immune checkpoint inhibitors either in combination (CTLA-4/PD-1) or as monotherapy, maculopapular eruption (50%) was the most common reaction. Among those who had any cutaneous reaction, a few (21%) of them were referred to dermatology.[63] There is 1 case report describing a patient with refractory acute lymphoblastic T-cell leukemia after allogeneic stem cell transplant who was treated with a PD-1 inhibitor. One week after administration, the patient developed acute graft-versus-host disease of the skin, liver, lung, central nervous system, and eyes.[64] Therefore, it is important to include graft-versus-host disease in the differential for an acute rash in a patient with a history of stem cell transplant who receives immunotherapy.

SUMMARY

- Targeted cancer therapies block specific molecular pathways involved in the growth, progression, and spread of cancer.
- Pediatric dermatology literature is emerging on the specific types and prevalence of cutaneous reactions to targeted therapies that hone in on membrane-bound receptors (eg, BCR-ABL, EGFR, or SMO inhibitors), intracellular signaling targets (eg, BRAF, MEK, mTOR), and antiangiogenesis agents (eg, VEGF), as well as targeted immunotherapies.
- Data regarding the timing, severity, and treatment algorithm for these cutaneous reactions are most plentiful for BRAF, MEK, and EGFR inhibitors.
- Further research on the most common cutaneous reactions of targeted therapy in children, treatments, and prevention is crucial to better serve the needs of this population.

CLINICS CARE POINTS

- Targeted cancer therapies induce a variable range of cutaneous toxicities that can be dose-limiting. Most common reactions in targeted therapies include follicular rash and xerosis.
- Data about onset of cutaneous reaction in pediatric populations are lacking, but onset in adults is within weeks.
- Preventative measures should be considered before starting targeted therapies.
- Dermatologists should tailor management to the type and severity of the cutaneous reaction.

ACKNOWLEDGMENTS

Funding for this project was made possible by the Pediatric Dermatology Research Alliance (PeDRA)

REFERENCES

1. Liu L, Oza S, Hogan D, et al. Global, regional, and national causes of child mortality in 2000–13, with projections to inform post-2015 priorities: an updated systematic analysis. Lancet 2015;385(9966): 430–40.
2. Carlberg VM, Davies OMT, Brandling-Bennett HA, et al. Cutaneous reactions to pediatric cancer treatment part II: targeted therapy. Pediatr Dermatol 2021;38(1):18–30.

3. Targeted Therapy for Cancer - National Cancer Institute. 2014. Available at: https://www.cancer.gov/about-cancer/treatment/types/targeted-therapies. March 21, 2021.
4. Carofiglio F, Lopalco A, Lopedota A, et al. Bcr-Abl tyrosine kinase inhibitors in the treatment of pediatric CML. Int J Mol Sci 2020;21(12).
5. Belum VR, Washington C, Pratilas CA, et al. Dermatologic adverse events in pediatric patients receiving targeted anticancer therapies: a pooled analysis. Pediatr Blood Cancer 2015;62(5):798–806.
6. Geoerger B, Morland B, Ndiaye A, et al. Target-driven exploratory study of imatinib mesylate in children with solid malignancies by the Innovative Therapies for Children with Cancer (ITCC) European Consortium. Eur J Cancer 2009;45(13):2342–51.
7. Larson JSM. Severe periorbital edema secondary to imatinib mesylate for chronic myelogenous leukemia. Arch Ophthalmol 2007;125(7):985.
8. Drucker AM, Wu S, Busam KJ, et al. Rash with the multitargeted kinase inhibitors nilotinib and dasatinib: meta-analysis and clinical characterization. Eur J Haematol 2013;90(2):142–50.
9. Brazzelli V, Roveda E, Prestinari F, et al. Vitiligo-like lesions and diffuse lightening of the skin in a pediatric patient treated with imatinib mesylate: a noninvasive colorimetric assessment. Pediatr Dermatol 2006;23(2):175–8.
10. Mahon C, Purvis D, Laughton S, et al. Imatinib mesylate-induced pseudoporphyria in two children. Pediatr Dermatol 2014;31(5):603–7.
11. Albert CM, Davis JL, Federman N, et al. TRK fusion cancers in children: a clinical review and recommendations for screening. J Clin Oncol 2018;37(6):513–24.
12. Kheder ES, Hong DS. Emerging targeted therapy for tumors with NTRK fusion proteins. Clin Cancer Res 2018;24(23):5807–14.
13. Zhao X, Kotch C, Fox E, et al. NTRK fusions identified in pediatric tumors: the frequency, fusion partners, and clinical outcome. JCO Precis Oncol 2021;(5):204–14.
14. Laetsch TW, DuBois SG, Mascarenhas L, et al. Larotrectinib for paediatric solid tumours harbouring NTRK gene fusions: a multicentre, open-label, phase 1 study. Lancet Oncol 2018;19(5):705–14.
15. Trippett TM, Herzog C, Whitlock JA, et al. Phase I and pharmacokinetic study of cetuximab and irinotecan in children with refractory solid tumors: a study of the Pediatric Oncology Experimental Therapeutic Investigators' Consortium. J Clin Oncol 2009;27(30):5102–8.
16. Geoerger B, Hargrave D, Thomas F, et al. Innovative therapies for children with cancer pediatric phase I study of erlotinib in brainstem glioma and relapsing/refractory brain tumors. Neuro-Oncol. 2011;13(1):109–18.
17. Yalon M, Rood B, MacDonald TJ, et al. A feasibility and efficacy study of rapamycin and erlotinib for recurrent pediatric low-grade glioma (LGG). Pediatr Blood Cancer 2013;60(1):71–6.
18. Fakih M, Vincent M. Adverse events associated with anti-EGFR therapies for the treatment of metastatic colorectal cancer. Curr Oncol 2010;17(Suppl 1):S18–30.
19. Lacouture ME, Anadkat M, Jatoi A, et al. Dermatologic toxicity occurring during anti-EGFR monoclonal inhibitor therapy in patients with metastatic colorectal cancer: a systematic review. Clin Colorectal Cancer 2018;17(2):85–96.
20. Lacouture ME, Mitchell EP, Piperdi B, et al. Skin toxicity evaluation protocol with panitumumab (STEPP), a phase II, open-label, randomized trial evaluating the impact of a pre-emptive skin treatment regimen on skin toxicities and quality of life in patients with metastatic colorectal cancer. J Clin Oncol 2010;28(8):1351–7.
21. Lupu I, Voiculescu V, Bacalbasa N, et al. Cutaneous adverse reactions specific to epidermal growth factor receptor inhibitors. J Med Life 2015;8(Spec Issue):57–61.
22. McMillan R, Matsui W. Molecular pathways: the hedgehog signaling pathway in cancer. Clin Cancer Res 2012;18(18):4883–8.
23. Gorlin RJ, Goltz RW. Multiple nevoid basal-cell epithelioma, jaw cysts and bifid rib. N Engl J Med 1960;262(18):908–12.
24. Kieran MW, Chisholm J, Casanova M, et al. Phase I study of oral sonidegib (LDE225) in pediatric brain and solid tumors and a phase II study in children and adults with relapsed medulloblastoma. Neuro-Oncol. 2017;19(11):1542–52.
25. Vismodegib in treating younger patients with recurrent or refractory medulloblastoma - study results - ClinicalTrials.gov. Available at: https://clinicaltrials.gov/ct2/show/results/NCT01239316. March 20, 2021.
26. Boull CL, Gardeen S, Abdali T, et al. Cutaneous reactions in children treated with MEK inhibitors, BRAF inhibitors, or combination therapy: a multicenter study. J Am Acad Dermatol 2020. https://doi.org/10.1016/j.jaad.2020.07.044.
27. Song H, Zhong CS, Kieran MW, et al. Cutaneous reactions to targeted therapies in children with CNS tumors: a cross-sectional study. Pediatr Blood Cancer 2019;66(6):e27682.
28. Lacouture ME, Duvic M, Hauschild A, et al. Analysis of dermatologic events in vemurafenib-treated patients with melanoma. Oncologist 2013;18(3):314–22.
29. Rogers HA, Estranero J, Gudka K, et al. The therapeutic potential of targeting the PI3K pathway in pediatric brain tumors. Oncotarget 2016;8(2):2083–95.

30. Jiang N, Dai Q, Su X, et al. Role of PI3K/AKT pathway in cancer: the framework of malignant behavior. Mol Biol Rep 2020;47(6):4587–629.
31. Safety, tolerability, efficacy and pharmacokinetics of copanlisib in pediatric patients - no study results posted - ClinicalTrials.gov. Available at: https://clinicaltrials.gov/ct2/show/results/NCT03458728. March 20, 2021.
32. National Cancer Institute (NCI). NCI-COG pediatric MATCH (molecular analysis for therapy choice)- phase 2 subprotocol of LY3023414 in patients with solid tumors. clinicaltrials.gov. 2021. Available at: https://clinicaltrials.gov/ct2/show/NCT03213678. March 18, 2021.
33. Keppler-Noreuil KM, Sapp JC, Lindhurst MJ, et al. Pharmacodynamic study of miransertib in individuals with proteus syndrome. Am J Hum Genet 2019;104(3):484–91.
34. Fouladi M, Perentesis JP, Phillips CL, et al. A phase I trial of MK-2206 in children with refractory malignancies: a Children's Oncology Group Study. Pediatr Blood Cancer 2014;61(7):1246–51.
35. Morgenstern DA, Marzouki M, Bartels U, et al. Phase I study of vinblastine and sirolimus in pediatric patients with recurrent or refractory solid tumors. Pediatr Blood Cancer 2014;61(1):128–33.
36. Davies M, Saxena A, Kingswood JC. Management of everolimus-associated adverse events in patients with tuberous sclerosis complex: a practical guide. Orphanet J Rare Dis 2017;12(1):35.
37. Peterson DE, O'Shaughnessy JA, Rugo HS, et al. Oral mucosal injury caused by mammalian target of rapamycin inhibitors: emerging perspectives on pathobiology and impact on clinical practice. Cancer Med 2016;5(8):1897–907.
38. Fidan K, Kandur Y, Sozen H, et al. How often do we face side effects of sirolimus in pediatric renal transplantation? Transplant Proc 2013;45(1):185–9.
39. Hymes LC, Warshaw BL. Five-year experience using sirolimus-based, calcineurin inhibitor-free immunosuppression in pediatric renal transplantation. Pediatr Transplant 2011;15(4):437–41.
40. Hammer J, Seront E, Duez S, et al. Sirolimus is efficacious in treatment for extensive and/or complex slow-flow vascular malformations: a monocentric prospective phase II study. Orphanet J Rare Dis 2018;13. https://doi.org/10.1186/s13023-018-0934-z.
41. Glade-Bender J, Kandel JJ, Yamashiro DJ. VEGF blocking therapy in the treatment of cancer. Expert Opin Biol Ther 2003;3(2):263–76.
42. Carmeliet P. VEGF as a key mediator of angiogenesis in cancer. Oncology 2005;69(Suppl. 3):4–10.
43. Barone A, Rubin JB. Opportunities and challenges for successful use of bevacizumab in pediatrics. Front Oncol 2013;3. https://doi.org/10.3389/fonc.2013.00092.
44. Pasquale MDD, Castellano A, Sio LD, et al. Bevacizumab in pediatric patients: how safe is it? Anticancer Res 2011;31(11):3953–7.
45. Turner DC, Navid F, Daw NC, et al. Population pharmacokinetics of bevacizumab in children with osteosarcoma: implications for dosing. Clin Cancer Res 2014;20(10):2783–92.
46. Wheeler H, Black J, Webb S, et al. Dehiscence of corticosteroid-induced abdominal striae in a 14-year-old boy treated with bevacizumab for recurrent glioblastoma. J Child Neurol 2012;27(7):927–9.
47. Laugier O, Padovani L, Verschuur A, Gaudy-Marqueste C, André N. Necrotic ulcerated and bleeding striae distensae following bevacizumab in a palliative setting for gliobastomatosis cerebri. doi:10.3332/ecancer.2017.756
48. Kim A, Widemann BC, Krailo M, et al. Phase 2 trial of sorafenib in children and young adults with refractory solid tumors: a report from the Children's Oncology Group. Pediatr Blood Cancer 2015; 62(9):1562–6.
49. Sorafenib tosylate in treating younger patients with relapsed or refractory rhabdomyosarcoma, Wilms tumor, liver cancer, or thyroid cancer - study results - ClinicalTrials.gov. Available at: https://clinicaltrials.gov/ct2/show/results/NCT01502410. March 21, 2021.
50. Inaba H, Panetta JC, Pounds SB, et al. Sorafenib population pharmacokinetics and skin toxicities in children and adolescents with refractory/relapsed leukemia or solid tumor malignancies. Clin Cancer Res 2019;25(24):7320–30.
51. Kusari A, Borok J, Han AM, et al. Hand-foot-skin reaction related to use of the multikinase inhibitor sorafenib and hard orthotics. Pediatr Dermatol 2018; 35(4):e206–9.
52. NYU Langone Health. Phase II study of sorafenib in children and young adults with recurrent or progressive low-grade astrocytomas. clinicaltrials.gov. 2016. Available at: https://clinicaltrials.gov/ct2/show/NCT01338857. March 18, 2021.
53. Pfizer A. Phase I/II study of sunitinib in young patients with advanced gastrointestinal stromal tumor. clinicaltrials.gov. 2019. Available at: https://clinicaltrials.gov/ct2/show/results/NCT01396148. March 18, 2021.
54. Study of Sutent®/Sunitinib. SU11248) in subjects with NF-1 plexiform neurofibromas - study results - ClinicalTrials.gov. Available at: https://clinicaltrials.gov/ct2/show/results/NCT01402817. March 21, 2021.
55. Pazopanib Paediatric Phase II Trial Children's Oncology Group (COG) in solid tumors - study results - ClinicalTrials.gov. Available at: https://clinicaltrials.gov/ct2/show/results/NCT01956669. April 10, 2021.
56. Que Y, Liang Y, Zhao J, et al. Treatment-related adverse effects with pazopanib, sorafenib and sunitinib in patients with advanced soft tissue sarcoma: a

pooled analysis. Cancer Manag Res 2018;10: 2141–50.
57. Kim JH. The effect of urea cream on sorafenib-associated hand-foot skin reaction in patients with Korean hepatocellular carcinoma patients: multicenter, prospective randomized double-blind controlled study. clinicaltrials.gov. 2019. Available at: https://clinicaltrials.gov/ct2/show/NCT03212625. March 18, 2021.
58. Merchant MS, Wright M, Baird K, et al. Phase I clinical trial of ipilimumab in pediatric patients with advanced solid tumors. Clin Cancer Res 2016; 22(6):1364–70.
59. Phase 2 study of ipilimumab in children and adolescents (12 to < 18 years) with previously treated or untreated, unresectable stage III or stage IV malignant melanoma - study results - ClinicalTrials.gov. Available at: https://clinicaltrials.gov/ct2/show/results/NCT01696045. March 21, 2021.
60. Geoerger B, Bergeron C, Gore L, et al. Phase II study of ipilimumab in adolescents with unresectable stage III or IV malignant melanoma. Eur J Cancer 2017;86:358–63.
61. Davis KL, Fox E, Merchant MS, et al. Nivolumab in children and young adults with relapsed or refractory solid tumours or lymphoma (ADVL1412): a multicentre, open-label, single-arm, phase 1–2 trial. Lancet Oncol 2020;21(4):541–50.
62. Geoerger B, Kang HJ, Yalon-Oren M, et al. Pembrolizumab in paediatric patients with advanced melanoma or a PD-L1-positive, advanced, relapsed, or refractory solid tumour or lymphoma (KEYNOTE-051): interim analysis of an open-label, single-arm, phase 1–2 trial. Lancet Oncol 2020;21(1):121–33.
63. McCormack L, Thompson LL, Chang MS, et al. Cutaneous adverse events to immune checkpoint inhibitors in pediatric populations: a retrospective cohort study. J Am Acad Dermatol 2020. https://doi.org/10.1016/j.jaad.2020.11.033. S019096222033070X.
64. Boekstegers A-M, Blaeschke F, Schmid I, et al. MRD response in a refractory paediatric T-ALL patient through anti-programmed cell death 1 (PD-1) Ab treatment associated with induction of fatal GvHD. Bone Marrow Transplant 2017;52(8):1221–4.

Laser Surgery for Dermatologic Conditions in Pediatric Patients

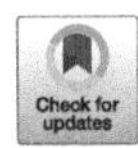

Deepti Gupta, MD

KEYWORDS

• Laser • Pediatric dermatology • Vascular • Pigmented lesion • Hidradenitis suppurativa
• Warts, Nevus of Ota

KEY POINTS

- Laser therapy is an effective treatment that can be used in a wide range of cutaneous conditions in pediatric dermatology.
- Real time tissue response to laser treatment can inform therapeutic effect, potential complications of the therapy, and whether parameter adjustments are necessary.
- The various make and models of lasers have different therapeutic settings that are not always generalizable across lasers of a specific wavelength.
- Safety precautions and type anesthesia are important considerations in pediatric patients.

INTRODUCTION

Laser is an acronym for light amplification by the stimulated emission of radiation. They have been widely used to treat various cutaneous disorders in pediatric dermatology. They are a valuable tool for pediatric dermatologists to have in their therapeutic toolbox as they can offer significant benefits with minimal morbidity. Lasers generate light of a specific wavelength by using energy in the form of an oscillating current to excite molecules within a certain media; solids (crystals), liquids (dyes), or gas (argon or CO2). As the current passes through one of these mediums the light that is discharged is coherent, meaning that the photos are precisely parallel (collimated) and aligned in both space and time. A coherent light can travel longer distances without attenuation. The wavelength of the laser is an important component of selective photothermolysis.[1] The longer the wavelength of the laser, generally the deeper the penetration of the energy. For wavelengths higher than 1064 nm the depth of penetration of the laser decreases as increased energy is dissipated into the surrounding tissue.

Lasers work through the concept of selective photothermolysis, allowing them to deliver energy very precisely based on the specific characteristics of the targeted tissue. The targeted chromophore and the size and depth of the lesion are the important characteristics of the tissue that help direct the appropriate laser wavelength choice to produce the most effective outcome. The 3 main chromophores within the tissue that absorb the energy of the laser are hemoglobin, melanin, and water. Chromophores have varying absorption spectrums and at select wavelengths, they have peaks in their absorption of the energy delivered by the laser. This allows for a more efficient transfer of energy to the targeted tissue, which minimizes tissue damage to the surrounding skin.

Selection of a laser

The selection of the specific wavelength of laser and parameters used is largely based on the following concepts:

1. Chromophore (considering the absorption spectrum and peaks of absorption)
2. Depth of the lesion
3. Size of the lesion

Department of Pediatrics, Division of Dermatology, Seattle Children's Hospital/University of Washington School of Medicine, 4800 Sand Point Way NE, PO BOX 5371, OC 9.834, Seattle, WA 98105, USA
E-mail address: Deepti.Gupta@seattlechildrens.org

Dermatol Clin 40 (2022) 215–225
https://doi.org/10.1016/j.det.2022.01.002
0733-8635/22/© 2022 Elsevier Inc. All rights reserved.

4. Individual characteristics of the patient (skin type, age, location being treated, and so forth)

Laser Types

There are 3 main categories of laser types; millisecond lasers, quality-switched (QS) laser, and ablative/nonablative lasers (**Table 1**). The concepts surrounding the millisecond and QS lasers have to do with pulse duration. The pulse duration, also known as the pulse width, is the time in which a targeted tissue is exposed to laser energy. A key factor in determining optimal pulse duration is thermal relaxation time. Thermal relaxation time refers to the time that it takes a photon to heat and then cool. In general, the larger the diameter of the target (ie, vessel, melanosome, pigmented molecule) within the tissue is longer the pulse duration. Millisecond lasers tend to target vascular lesions with larger diameter targets than quality-switched (QS) lasers that target very small tattoo particles or pigment granules within melanosomes. The chromophore of millisecond lasers is oxyhemoglobin and QS lasers is melanin. The specific type of laser chosen not only has to do with the type of tissue being targeted, but also with the depth of the lesion. The longer the wavelength, the deeper the laser energy will penetrate. The third category of lasers is ablative and nonablative lasers that target water as their chromophore. Ablative means that the laser vaporizes or ablates the area treated to destroy or remove the tissue completely. Nonablative lasers on the other hand transfer energy to injure the tissue through melting or coagulating the tissue. Both of these modes activate tissue healing to improve the skin texture. The ablative and nonablative lasers can further be fractionated, meaning that instead of fully ablating an area, the tissue is broken up into adjacent zones of normal tissue and treated tissue in a checkerboard pattern. Fractionated lasers have quicker recovery times than fully ablative laser treatments due to the fact that normal tissue is sitting adjacent to the treated areas allowing remodeling of tissue to occur more rapidly.

Laser devices

It should be noted that lasers of a specific wavelength come in different models and brands and have different parameters for the treatment of similar conditions. Therefore, it is difficult to extrapolate published laser settings to all lasers within even a specific wavelength. Treatment protocols vary by device; therefore, understanding the laser-specific treatment's parameters for your device and expected versus dangerous tissue response endpoints, are an important guide therapy.

Laser safety

Eye safety is of the utmost importance for the patient and all individuals in the laser treatment room.[2] The surgeon should call out before the procedure the appropriate glasses to wear with the wavelength corresponding to the laser being used, color of glasses, and ensure all in the room have eye protection. Individuals in the laser room should also check glasses to ensure the wavelength of laser people used in appropriate for their glasses. Depending on the treatment site, the patient should be protected with either opaque eye pads (if lasering the face), metal corneal eye shields (if lasering around the eye), or if the treated area is not on the face and depending on the age/cooperation of the patient, it may be possible for them to wear laser goggles if proper fit and compliance are assured. Cotton or adhesive laser-safe eye pads, when treating very young children, are often held in place during the procedure by a member of the treatment team. When treating within the orbital rim, a metal corneal eye shield should be placed with anesthetic eye drops and nonflammable lubricant eye gel to avoid corneal abrasions.

Using a smoke evacuator and appropriate masks for all in the room is also important during procedures. Reports of viral plume present in the air after the laser treatment of warts, especially with the use of CO2 lasers.[3] Risk of infection with human papillomavirus was greatest with treating genital warts.[4] Surgical masks have been effective in decreasing the risk of HPV infection to surgeon and staff. There have also been reports documenting the release of hazardous and ultrafine particles after laser hair removal procedures into the air and having ill effects on health.[5,6] In addition, the smell of charring skin and hair can be uncomfortable to patients and staff in the treatment room. The use of smoke evacuators has been shown to be effective at clearing the release of these nanoparticles when used during laser procedures of hair-bearing areas. It is recommended that smoke evacuators be used for the safety of all surgeons and staff during laser hair removal procedures.[7]

Anesthesia considerations

There are a variety of anesthesia options that can be used with laser therapy. Pretreatment with topical amide anesthetics such as topical lidocaine or prilocaine, use of oral pain medications such as acetaminophen and nonsteroidal anti-inflammatories, or intra-nasal or oral anxiolytic medications are options depending on the clinical context and setting. Nonsteroidal anti-inflammatories should be avoided when treating

Table 1
Laser types

Millisecond Lasers	Quality-Switched Lasers	Ablative	Nonablative
Pulsed Dye Laser (595 nm)	Quality-Switched KTP/ Frequency-doubled Nd Yag (532 nm)	Carbon Dioxide (CO2) (10,600 nm)	Erbium: Glass (1540 nm)
Potassium Titanyl Phosphate (KTP)/ Long-pulsed frequency-doubled Nd Yag (532 nm)	Quality-Switched Ruby (694 nm)	Erbium-yttrium argon garnet (Er:YAG) (2,940 nm)	
Long-Pulsed Alexandrite Laser (755 nm)	Quality-Switched Alexandrite (755 nm)		
Long-Pulsed Diode Laser (800–810, 940, 980 nm)	Quality-Switched Long-pulsed Nd Yag (1064 nm)		
Long-Pulsed Nd Yag Laser (1064 nm)			

vascular lesions. Injectable anesthetics can also be used to perform nerve blocks to anesthetize areas before the use of ablative and nonablative lasers or deeper-penetrating lasers such as LP Nd Yag.

During laser treatment, gate control theory has been used by applying pressure directly to the skin or tapping the skin to activate pressure receptors and diminish pain response from laser treatment by having a decrease in pain sensation travel to the central nervous system. The gate control theory of pain describes how using nonpainful sensations to activate tactile and pressure skin receptors can naturally block the transmission of pain to the brain during the laser procedure.[8] In addition, skin cooling via cryogen spray, direct cooling tip within the laser, or forced cooling air have also been used to decrease intraoperative pain. As an adjuvant to anesthesia, distraction techniques can also be used to help mitigate pain and discomfort. During laser cases music, tactile and sensory tools such as the use of stress balls or fidget objects, and use of screens when patients able to safely use laser glasses can be used.

General anesthesia in the operating room under the guidance of trained anesthesiologists can also be used when needed. Currently limited studies and FDA warning have discussed the potential neurocognitive effects associated with anesthesia in young children, especially with repeated anesthesia events in patients under the age of 3 years.[9] When selecting the correct anesthesia mode for a patient, shared decision-making should be used, and a discussion of potential risks and benefits should be had with patients and families.

Monitoring tissue response and evaluation of clinical endpoints

The clinical endpoint is observed intraoperatively and allows the laser surgeon to gauge the therapeutic effect of the laser treatment. The surgeon is able to assess whether laser settings are correct to achieve the desired endpoint or if any fine-tuning of laser parameters are needed. Laser settings such as energy/fluence, spot size, and pulse duration can be changed based on observed clinical endpoints. Some tissue responses are seen immediately, while others may take a few minutes to become visible. The desired clinical endpoints and those that can be signs of tissue damage and should be avoided vary by the type of laser being used and the chromophore being targeted. These endpoints are outlined in **Table 2**.

Procedural considerations

- Preprocedure:
  - Strict sun protection starting at least 6 to 8 weeks before the procedure to reduce competing epidermal melanin content
  - Assess infection risk (highest with HSV infections and with ablative laser resurfacing, the risk still low at approximately 5% of procedures, nonablative procedures 0.6% risk) and start antiviral for Herpes labialis prophylaxis treatment 1 day before laser procedure in those at high risk.

Table 2
Tissue response and clinical endpoints

Chromophore (Target)	Lasers Used	Desired Clinical Endpoint	Signs of Tissue Injury
Hemoglobin	PDL, KTP, Alexandrite,	Purpura, vessel darkening, vessel disappearance	Gray or white coloration of the tissue; blistering or positive Nikolsky sign (late)
Hemoglobin	LP Nd Yag	Erythema (may take a few minutes to develop), vessel darkening, or vessel contraction	Gray or white coloration of the tissue; blistering
Hemoglobin (warts)	PDL, LP Nd Yag	Intense purpura	Blister, scar
Melanin (laser hair removal)	LP Ruby, LP Alexandrite, LP Nd Yag	Perifollicular erythema and edema, erythema (delayed response, may take up to 5 min to be visible)	Dyspigmentation (late)
Melanin and dermal pigmentation	Q-switched Ruby, Q-switched Alexandrite, Q-switched Nd Yag	Frosting, superficial whitening, and auditory snap or crack	Dyspigmentation (late)

- Postprocedure:
  - Cold compresses and ice used for 24 to 48 hours after the laser procedure
  - Petrolatum-based ointment is recommended immediately postop and until the area is completely healed.
  - Protect site treated from friction and trauma
  - Typically patients can return to school and daily activities on the same day or within 2 to 3 days of laser treatment depending on laser, site, and surface area treated
  - Compression garments can be helpful to reduce laser-induced postoperative edema (ie, treatment of venous malformations (VM))
  - Sun protection and avoidance of direct sun exposure
  - Use of adjuvant treatments such as topical rapamycin should start immediately after laser treatment
  - Oral antihistamines and topical steroid ointment may be recommended for patients who develop immediate urticarial reactions to laser treatment

DISEASE-SPECIFIC LASER TREATMENT

Laser treatment of vascular lesions

Lasers are widely used and often considered first-line treatment of many vascular lesions. The chromophore for vascular lesions is oxyhemoglobin, which has the greatest absorption peaks at 418, 542, 577 nm. The energy from the laser is absorbed by oxyhemoglobin and this heat energy is then transferred to the wall of the vessel, causing the destruction of the vessel by coagulation and closure or leakage of the vessel. For many vascular lesions, the PDL laser (585–600 nm; 595 nm most common) is most often used. The PDL penetrates to a maximum depth of 1.2 mm. Deoxyhemoglobin is another chromophore within vascular lesions that can be targeted. This is the chromophore of choice within VM and refractory and hypertrophic port-wine birthmarks (PWB), with its absorption peak near 750 nm and 930 nm. For deoxyhemoglobin, the Alexandrite laser (755 nm) and Long-pulsed Nd Yag laser (1064 nm) have been used as their wavelengths more closely align with the absorption peaks of deoxyhemoglobin.

Port-wine birthmarks

Port-wine birthmarks (PWB) are largely congenital vascular malformations that are present at birth and comprised of ectatic capillaries and postcapillary venules within the superficial vascular plexus. PWB were previously referred to as "port wine stains," but the term stain holds a negative connotation and therefore the preferred term is PWB.[10] PWB are persistent and grow proportionally with the patient. PWB can become darker, hypertrophic, nodular, develop vascular pyogenic granuloma-like blebs, and can have associated soft-tissue overgrowth due to progressive vascular ectasia and enlargement of the diameter of vessels.[11] The size of the vessels can vary significantly within PWB from 7 to 300 μm, with larger vessel size in adults and in darker PWB. Laser treatment of PWB is aimed to decrease these effects, as well as reduce psycho-social burden on patients and families.

Pulsed dye laser has been effective in treating PWB in patients of all skin types, but the individual response is variable. Therapeutic effect is based on many factors such as size and depth of lesion, location, and individual characteristics such as skin pigmentation and age. Approximately 20% of patients experience complete clearance and 80% have a decrease in color and thickness of their PWB.[12] In darker-skinned individuals with dynamic cooling, clearance rates and effectiveness of PDL was also favorable.[13,14] Predictors of more favorable treatment outcomes include small size (<20 cm^2), location over bony areas such as the central forehead whereby the depth of the skin is thinner, and initiation of early treatment (<6 months of age).[15] Early initiation of therapy has shown greater rates of clearance with infants who initiated therapy before 6 months of age were noted to have rates of clearance close to 90% after 1 year of treatment.[16] Early treatment is thought to be effective for a variety of reasons. In younger patients, the skin is thinner, which allows for better penetration of the laser to ectatic capillaries at varying depths. There is less melanin present in younger patients which not only causes less side effects from the laser, but there is also less uptake of energy in the surrounding tissues due to less competition for the laser target. Hemoglobin F is present in infants which allows for an additional target for laser therapy. Finally, the diameter or the dilation of lesional vessels is decreased in younger individuals making them more amenable to laser treatment.

Treatment intervals vary and have been documented from 2 to 6 weeks. Recent meta-analysis and systemic review of the literature demonstrated that time intervals between PDL treatments were not associated with PWB outcomes, but younger age at intervention, light Fitzpatrick skin type, and facial location were associated with increased improvement rates.[17] Multiple treatments are often required to achieve clearance or a plateau in response. Often 10 or more treatments have proven to be beneficial. Typically, the desired tissue endpoint with pulsed dye laser is immediate purpura; however, purpura may be delayed if larger spot sizes are used. If laser fluence is too high there can be a gray to white color or blistering of the skin. This endpoint is not always immediately evident and indicates epidermal injury that may not be reversible and may lead to scarring. Therefore, careful monitoring of tissue response—purpura, edema, blistering—is incredibly important intraoperatively in areas immediately being lasered as well as those that have just been lasered.

Bruising (purpura) and mild swelling of the treated areas are expected outcomes after laser and may last 1 to 2 weeks after treatment. Hyper or hypopigmentation of the tissue may also occur and is often transient. Darker-skinned individuals are more at risk for skin dyspigmentation after laser treatment which may last longer. Complications of pulsed dye laser treatment may occur when treating hair-bearing areas, especially in dark-haired individuals, as there can be a decrease in hair or permanent hair loss. This can occur more often in younger children and in areas whereby skin is thinner such as the eyebrow and overlying bony prominences. Redarkening of the PWB can occur after lightning with laser treatment. The redarkened areas are often still improved and lighter in appearance than the original PWB.[18]

The settings used for an individual depend on a multitude of factors specific to the patient and equipment being used. Patient-specific factors include patient age, location of treatment, intensity of lesional color, number of treatments performed, and skin color. Specific equipment parameters such as make and model of laser device, age of machine, recent maintenance of laser can also all effect laser settings selected. Settings can vary greatly and therefore can be difficult to extrapolate from one laser type to another or from the literature, even if the laser is of the same wavelength. Therefore, the suggested laser settings from the literature are provided with their references with these words of caution, and advice to monitor tissue response and clinical endpoints.

Proposed settings for the treatment of PWB are 7 to 10 mm spot size, 8 to 12 J/cm^2, pulse duration of 0.45 to 6 ms, and cooling with a burst of cryogen spray of 20 to 30 ms with a 30 ms delay between the end of the cryogen spray and repeat firing of the laser. In darker-skinned individuals use of dynamic cooling has minimized side effects from laser treatment, but also using longer pulse duration/pulse width, larger spot size, and initiating treatment at a lower fluence may be appropriate to decrease potential side effects of the laser such as hypo or hyper-pigmentation and scarring.[13,14] In one study in Indian patients, Fitzpatrick skin type IV to V settings proposed were; spot size 7 to 10 mm and depending on situation 0.45 ms at 6.5–8 J/cm^2, 1.5 ms at 8 to 12 J/cm^2, 3 ms at 8 to

12 J/cm², and 10 ms at 10 to 15 J/cm².[13] For infants, laser parameters may also have lower fluences due to thinner epidermis, and smaller pulse durations due to decreased caliber and dilatation of ectatic vessels. To deliver even pulses throughout the entire lesion it is recommended that there be a 10% to 30% overlap between the pulses. "Stacking" of pulses should be avoided as it may lead to more adverse effects. The laser should also be held perpendicular to the skin being treated to prevent epidermal injury in the shape of an arcuate epidermal burn due to a misallignment in contact of the laser and cryogen cooling spray with the skin.[19]

REFRACTORY PORT-WINE BIRTHMARKS

PWB that are refractory to pulsed dye laser treatment may benefit from a longer wavelength laser (Alexandrite, 755 nm) or a combined approach with shorter and longer wavelength lasers (PDL + LP Nd Yag) to target deeper and larger caliber ectatic vessels. These lasers have a 50% to 75% increase in-depth that they can penetrate. Suggested laser parameters for Alexandrite laser for refractory PWB are spot size 8 to 12 mm, pulse duration 3 ms, cryogen spray of 40 to 60 ms with a 40 ms delay, and fluence range of 35 to 100 J/cm² with most fluences between 60 and 85 J/cm².[20] Caution is advised, as longer wavelength lasers, especially LP Nd Yag,[21] have narrower therapeutic windows and have a higher risk of adverse effects, such as deep thermal burns and scarring; therefore, they should be carefully selected with shared decision with family and patient. Additional treatments have been described such as using adjuvant posttreatment anti-angiogenesis agents such as topical rapamycin, an mTOR inhibitor that inhibits angiogenesis induced by laser vessel damage.[22] Rapamycin has been shown to be beneficial in some patients and clinical trials, but has not been universally effective.[23] One proposed treatment regimen includes treatment with once-a-day topical application of 1% rapamycin for up to 12 weeks following laser treatment.[24]

Spider angiomas

Spider angiomas (SA) are benign telangiectasias that have a central feeder vessel with fine dilated radiating vessels branching outward from the center. They are common and occur in approximately 10% to 15% of healthy children and adults. Various laser treatments have been described, with pulsed dye laser being the most common. PDL has been shown to be an effective laser to treat SA with clearance noted to be near 90% after 1 treatment and 91% after 2 treatments,[25] but KTP and intense pulsed light (IPL) laser have also been used effectively to treat SA.[26,27] Treatment parameters are as follows: PDL, 595 nm, spot size 7 mm, Fluence 40 J/cm², pulse duration of 3 ms, 30/20 cooling.[25] PDL settings can be adjusted to account for smaller spot size depending in the size of lesions and small pulse duration due to caliber of telangiectasia. If either of these settings is adjusted the fluence will also need to be adjusted. KTP 532 nm, spot size 2 mm, 10 to 12 J/cm², pulse duration of 10 to 14 ms[26] and IPL with cooling tip 550 nm, 25 to 27 J/cm² and 5 ms pulse duration.[27]Of note, when using IPL, the handpiece is often much too large for the size of the SA; therefore, a cover should be used to protect unaffected skin.

Infantile hemangiomas

Infantile hemangiomas are benign vascular tumors that derive from the proliferations of endothelial cells. A majority of infantile hemangiomas do not require treatment, but a minority due to functional impairment, disfigurement/risk of disfigurement, or ulceration. The use of propranolol, a beta-blocker medication, is considered first-line therapy for large or complex lesions. Laser can be a play a primary role for small and relatively flat lesions,[28] and an adjuvant role to beta-blocker treatment. Early treatment of infantile hemangiomas can prevent growth and accelerate the transition to plateau or involution phase and decrease disfigurement.[29] Suggested laser settings 595 nm, 10 mm spot, Fluence 7.75 to 9.5 J cm,² pulse duration 1.5 ms, dynamic cooling 30/20[16]. When treating infantile hemangiomas low fluences were used and would recommend against any stacking or overlap of pulses due to risk of ulceration, PDL laser treatment in combination with Propranolol[30] and used in combination with timolol[31] were shown to be more effective than monotherapy with any one treatment modality. Pulsed dye laser can also be used for the treatment of ulcerated hemangiomas (suggested laser settings 595 nm, 10 mm spot, Fluence 5–7 J cm,² pulse duration 1.5 ms, dynamic cooling 30/20) and for the residual telangiectasias and fibrofatty residua[32] (Suggested settings, CO2 fractionated ablative laser, 5%–10% density, 20 mJ) of involuted hemangiomas. Hemangioma skin can be more vulnerable to erosion, ulceration, and scarring after laser treatment than capillary malformations, so caution is advised and conservative parameters are recommended when treating hemangiomas with laser.

Angiofibromas

Angiofibromas are erythematous papules located on the central face. They can occur as isolated lesions, or more commonly arise as a cutaneous manifestation of tuberous sclerosis. Angiofibromas are one of the earlier signs of tuberous sclerosis and can begin to appear as early as 2 to 5 years of age. Angiofibromas can be treated with pulsed dye laser, KTP laser, as well as CO2 ablative fractionated laser. KTP and PDL (suggested settings 595 nm, 10 mm spot, 7.5–9 J/cm^2, 1.5 ms pulse duration, 30/20 dynamic cooling)[33] laser treatments are more effective with smaller and more vascular appearing angiofibromas, while CO2 (10,600 nm, 5 mm spot, 0.1-second repeat, fluence 125 mJ/3.5 W, 5%–6% density) laser can be more effective for larger (>4 mm) and less vascular appearing angiofibromas. Laser treatment can be used in combination with, topical rapamycin, an mTOR inhibitor, which has been shown to be effective in treating and preventing further angiofibromas in TS.

Venous malformations and glomuvenous malformations

VM (VM) and glomuvenous malformations (GVM) are congenital vascular birthmarks that are not always apparent at birth. Over time they increase in size and can be complicated by pain secondary to thrombosis, swelling, and erythema. GVM develop in new locations over time are more superficially located and can be quite painful. There are various treatment modalities that can be used for VM including sclerotherapy, excision, glue excision,[34] medical treatment, and laser surgery. Laser can be used as a monotherapy or in conjunction with other treatment modalities. The laser should be chosen based on the depth of the VM or GVM, with shorter wavelengths, PDL, used for more superficial VMs and Alexandrite (755 nm, spot size 3 mm, 44 J/cm^2) and LP Nd Yag (1064 nm, 4–6 mm spot size, pulse duration 25–40 ms, fluence 35–70 J/cm^2) laser used for nodular VMs, VMs located in the dermis or subcutaneous fat, or GVMs. Alexandrite and LP Nd Yag lasers[35,36] can be used in combination with PDL and it is recommended that laser pulses have minimal overlap.

Lymphatic malformations

Lymphatic malformations (LMs) are congenital vascular anomalies comprised of malformed, dilated, and disorganized lymphatic channels. LMs can be characterized as macrocystic, microcystic, or combined. Treatment of LMs can be conducted with LP Nd Yag and LP Alexandrite lasers especially if there is a hemorrhagic component present within the blebs. CO2 (10,600 nm, ablative fractionated laser, 25 mJ, 2 passes, 10% density)[37,38] ablative laser may also be used in cases whereby there is a lack of a hemorrhagic component to target.

Laser treatment for pigmented lesions

Becker nevus

Becker nevus (BN) is an organoid hamartoma characterized by a segmental area of hyperpigmentation and hypertrichosis most commonly located over the shoulder, chest, and scapula. It often appears in adolescence, but congenital cases have been described. Laser treatments are aimed at either hyperpigmentation, using QS lasers or fractionated ablative lasers, or hypertrichosis using laser hair removal devices which are generally Alexandrite (755 nm) or Diode (810 nm) for individuals with lighter hair and LP Nd Yag (1064 nm) for individuals with darker hair.[39]

Melanocytic nevi

The removal of melanocytic nevi in children with laser therapy is controversial and is generally not recommended.

Congenital melanocytic nevi

Laser treatment for the removal of Congenital Melanocytic Nevi (CMN) is also not recommended. However, laser hair removal has been reported to be effective for the treatment of hypertrichosis with a CMN. The cutaneous features of a CMN with increased nodularity and rugosity can make it difficult to shave or precisely clip the hair, therefore, making laser hair removal an effective option. There have not been any reports of malignant transformation of the CMN after laser hair removal techniques.[40] The final coloration of the CMN also does not seem to be altered by laser treatment.[41]

Nevus of Ota/Nevus of Ito

Nevus of Ota and Nevus of Ito are forms of dermal melanocytosis located specifically around the eye and face in Nevus of Ota and along the arm/shoulder for Nevus of Ito. The QS lasers have been effective in treating these conditions and early treatment is associated with better results.[42,43] If treating within the orbital rim a metal corneal eye shield will need to be placed with topical ophthalmic anesthetic drops and nonflammable lubricating gel.

Laser treatment for other conditions

Keratosis pilaris rubra

Keratosis pilaris (KP) is a common skin condition characterized by follicular plugging affecting the cheeks, lateral arms, and proximal thighs. It is often accompanied or background erythema, termed Keratosis Pilaris Rubra (KPR). Treatment of KPR is

Table 3
Indication for use of lasers in pediatric dermatology

Laser Type (Wavelength nm)	Target (Chromophore)	Indication	Expected Endpoint
Excimer (308 nm)	Nonspecific	Vitiligo, Psoriasis, Atopic Dermatitis, Alopecia Areata	None
KTP Long Pulsed (532 nm)	Hemoglobin	Angiofibroma, Spider angioma, Telangiectasias	Disappearance of the vessel, coagulation of the vessel or lesion
KTP QS (532 nm)	Melanin	Café au lait macules, ephelides	Immediate whitening
Pulsed Dye Laser (585–600 nm; 595 nm most common)	Hemoglobin	• Vascular lesions: Port wine birthmarks, facial telangiectasias, spider angiomas, Infantile hemangiomas • Keratosis Pilaris Rubra Erythematous scars/ striae • Warts	Purpura, vessel disappearance, vessel darkening
Long-Pulsed Ruby (694 nm)	Melanin	Hair removal	Erythema, mild perifollicular edema
QS Ruby (694 nm)	Melanin	Nevus of Ota/Ito, dermal pigment	Immediate whitening
Long-Pulsed Alexandrite (755 nm)	Hemoglobin	Hypertrophic or PDL refractory PWB, laser hair removal	Purpura after 5 min or more (PWB), erythema and perifollicular erythema (hair removal)
QS Alexandrite (755 nm)	Melanin	Nevus of Ota/Ito, dermal pigment, café au lait, Becker's nevus	Immediate whitening
Diode (800 nm)	Deoxyhemoglobin	Hair removal	Erythema, mild erythema, and perifollicular erythema (hair removal)
Long-Pulsed Nd Yag (1064 nm)	Deoxyhemoglobin, Melanin	Hair removal, venous malformations, glomuvenous malformations, PDL resistant PWB and hypertrophic PWB, warts	
QS Nd Yag (1064 nm)	Melanin	Nevus of Ota/Ito, dermal pigment, Becker's nevus	
Erb: Yag (2940 nm)	Water	Ablation of epidermal lesions, skin resurfacing, scars, acne scarring	Pinpoint columns of destruction (fractionated); Full-field ablation
CO2 (10,600 nm)	Water	Ablation of epidermal lesions, skin resurfacing, scars, acne scarring	Pinpoint columns of destruction (fractionated); Full-field ablation

Adapted from Lehmer and Kelly "Laser surgery" Procedural Pediatric Dermatology, Edition 1[48–50].

often disappointing with the use of topical emollients, topical keratolytics, topical retinoids, and topical anti-inflammatory agents such as topical calcineurin inhibitors and topical corticosteroids that have shown little effect for the erythema. There have been case series looking at laser treatment of KPR.[44] For maintenance of results treatment must be continued or lesions and the erythema will often occur. Out of all laser treatments discussed in the literature, pulsed dye laser has been shown to be most effective with longer lasting improvement and decrease in recurrence. Suggested laser settings with PDL, 595 nm, spot size 7 to 10 mm, fluence 4.5 to 11.5 J/cm^2 (most treated with 8–11.5 J/m^2), pulse duration ranged from 1.5 to 10 msec (most treated with a pulse duration of 1.5 or 3 msec), and dynamic cooling 30/20[44].

HIDRADENITIS SUPPURATIVA

Hidradenitis suppurativa (HS) is a chronic follicular disease that causes painful inflammation, scarring, draining nodular and sinus tracts with predilection for intertriginous areas. Most patients present after puberty. There is a broad range of medical and surgical therapies for HS. Laser hair removal works best as adjuvant therapy and has been effective by causing follicular destruction. Primary endpoints observed for the laser include perifollicular erythema and edema. The scarring sinus tracts are not effectively treated with laser, but individuals with recurrent nodules and abscesses, which tend to be a marker of active follicular disease, tend to have the best results from laser therapy. The treatments focus on destroying hair follicles and debulking lesions through ablation. A variety of lasers have been described in the treatment of HS including LP Nd Yag, IPL, Alexandrite, Diode, and CO2 ablative lasers.[45]

WARTS

Warts are caused by human papillomavirus (HPV). Laser treatment is one therapy that can be used for recalcitrant warts. Pairing the wart before the procedure makes the laser procedure more effective. Application of topical lidocaine before treatment makes the treatment more tolerable and can also make paring of the wart easier by softening the wart. In addition to laser-appropriate eye protection, a smoke evacuator and a surgical or charcoal mask should be used for laser due to the potential aerosolization of HPV during the procedure.[4] Laser treatment with PDL (595 nm, spot size 5–7 mm, Fluence 9–14 J/cm^2, pulse duration 0.45–1.5 ms, no cooling for nonfacial warts) should include 1 to 2 mm of normal skin around the wart for the zone of treatment. LP Nd Yag laser can also be used for the treatment of warts (1064 nm, 3–6 mm spot size, 180–300 J/cm^2 pulse duration 20 ms, no cooling for nonfacial warts).[46] CO2 laser can also be used to treat warts. Both of the above-mentioned settings are for nonfacial warts and again the treatment parameters are difficult to apply to other laser machines. For the treatment of warts on the face, dynamic cooling is used and lower fluence and spot size matching size of the wart.[47] If the clinical endpoint of purpura is not achieved, up to 3 passes over the wart can be performed. Treatment can be repeated every 4 to 6 weeks.**Table 3**

CLINICS CARE POINTS

- Lasers can treat a wide variety of conditions within pediatric dermatology with significant benefit and limited morbidity
- Early initiation, less than 6 months of age, of laser treatment of PWB has improved outcomes
- Use of larger spot sizes, decreased fluence, dynamic cooling longer pulse durations can minimize adverse reactions to laser therapy for darker-skinned individuals.
- Laser settings cannot be generalizable across all device types for a specific wavelength of laser.
- Monitoring tissue response and clinical endpoints are important to assess the efficacy of the treatment and allow for intraoperative fine-tuning of laser parameters

DISCLOSURE

The authors have nothing to disclose.

REFERENCES

1. Anderson RR. Lasers in dermatology–a critical update. J Dermatol 2000;27(11):700–5.
2. Sliney DH. Laser safety. Lasers Surg Med 1995;16(3):215–25.
3. Sawchuk WS, Weber PJ, Lowy DR, et al. Infectious papillomavirus in the vapor of warts treated with carbon dioxide laser or electrocoagulation: detection and protection. J Am Acad Dermatol 1989;21(1):41–9.

4. Gloster HM Jr, Roenigk RK. Risk of acquiring human papillomavirus from the plume produced by the carbon dioxide laser in the treatment of warts. J Am Acad Dermatol 1995;32(3):436–41.
5. Chuang GS, Farinelli W, Christiani DC, et al. Gaseous and particulate content of laser hair removal plume. JAMA Dermatol 2016;152(12):1320–6.
6. Eshleman EJ, LeBlanc M, Rokoff LB, et al. Occupational exposures and determinants of ultrafine particle concentrations during laser hair removal procedures. Environ Health 2017;16(1):30.
7. Katoch S, Mysore V. Surgical smoke in dermatology: its hazards and management. J Cutan Aesthet Surg 2019;12(1):1–7.
8. Fournier N. Hair removal on dark-skinned patients with pneumatic skin flattening (PSF) and a high-energy Nd:YAG laser. J Cosmet Laser Ther 2008; 10(4):210–2.
9. Andropoulos DB, Greene MF. Anesthesia and developing brains - implications of the FDA Warning. N Engl J Med 2017;376(10):905–7.
10. Hagen SL, Grey KR, Korta DZ, et al. Quality of life in adults with facial port-wine stains. J Am Acad Dermatol 2017;76(4):695–702.
11. Geronemus RG, Ashinoff R. The medical necessity of evaluation and treatment of port-wine stains. J Dermatol Surg Oncol 1991;17(1):76–9.
12. Brightman LA, Geronemus RG, Reddy KK. Laser treatment of port-wine stains. Clin Cosmet Investig Dermatol 2015;8:27–33.
13. Thajudheen CP, Jyothy K, Priyadarshini A. Treatment of port-wine stains with flash lamp pumped pulsed dye laser on Indian skin: a six year study. J Cutan Aesthet Surg 2014;7(1):32–6.
14. Shi W, Wang J, Lin Y, et al. Treatment of port wine stains with pulsed dye laser: a retrospective study of 848 cases in Shandong Province, People's Republic of China. Drug Des Devel Ther 2014;8: 2531–8.
15. Nguyen CM, Yohn JJ, Huff C, et al. Facial port wine stains in childhood: prediction of the rate of improvement as a function of the age of the patient, size and location of the port wine stain and the number of treatments with the pulsed dye (585 nm) laser. Br J Dermatol 1998;138(5):821–5.
16. Chapas AM, Eickhorst K, Geronemus RG. Efficacy of early treatment of facial port wine stains in newborns: a review of 49 cases. Lasers Surg Med 2007;39(7):563–8.
17. Snast I, Lapidoth M, Kaftory R, et al. Does interval time between pulsed dye laser treatments for port-wine stains influence outcome? A systematic review and meta-analysis. Lasers Med Sci 2021;36(9): 1909–16.
18. Nelson JS, Geronemus RG. Redarkening of port-wine stains 10 years after laser treatment. N Engl J Med 2007;356(26):2745–6 [author reply: 2746].
19. Lee SJ, Park SG, Kang JM, et al. Cryogen-induced arcuate shaped hyperpigmentation by dynamic cooling device. J Eur Acad Dermatol Venereol 2008;22(7):883–4.
20. Izikson L, Nelson JS, Anderson RR. Treatment of hypertrophic and resistant port wine stains with a 755 nm laser: a case series of 20 patients. Lasers Surg Med 2009;41(6):427–32.
21. Alster TS, Tanzi EL. Combined 595-nm and 1,064-nm laser irradiation of recalcitrant and hypertrophic port-wine stains in children and adults. Dermatol Surg 2009;35(6):914–8 [discussion: 918-9].
22. Gao L, Phan S, Nadora DM, et al. Topical rapamycin systematically suppresses the early stages of pulsed dye laser-induced angiogenesis pathways. Lasers Surg Med 2014;46(9):679–88.
23. Bloom BS, Nelson JS, Geronemus RG. Topical rapamycin combined with pulsed dye laser (PDL) in the treatment of capillary vascular malformations-Anatomical differences in response to PDL are relevant to interpretation of study results. J Am Acad Dermatol 2015;73(2):e71.
24. Lipner SR. Topical adjuncts to pulsed dye laser for treatment of port wine stains: review of the literature. Dermatol Surg 2018;44(6):796–802.
25. Yang B, Li L, Zhang LX, et al. Clinical characteristics and treatment options of infantile vascular anomalies. Medicine (Baltimore) 2015;94(40):e1717.
26. Clark C, Cameron H, Moseley H, et al. Treatment of superficial cutaneous vascular lesions: experience with the KTP 532 nm laser. Lasers Med Sci 2004;19(1):1–5.
27. Srinivas CR, Kumaresan M. Lasers for vascular lesions: standard guidelines of care. Indian J Dermatol Venereol Leprol 2011;77(3):349–68.
28. Shen L, Zhou G, Zhao J, et al. Pulsed dye laser therapy for infantile hemangiomas: a systemic review and meta-analysis. QJM 2015;108(6):473–80.
29. Kwon SH, Choi JW, Byun SY, et al. Effect of early long-pulse pulsed dye laser treatment in infantile hemangiomas. Dermatol Surg 2014;40(4):405–11.
30. Reddy KK, Blei F, Brauer JA, et al. Retrospective study of the treatment of infantile hemangiomas using a combination of propranolol and pulsed dye laser. Dermatol Surg 2013;39(6):923–33.
31. Asilian A, Mokhtari F, Kamali AS, et al. Pulsed dye laser and topical timolol gel versus pulse dye laser in treatment of infantile hemangioma: a double-blind randomized controlled trial. Adv Biomed Res 2015;4:257.
32. Brauer JA, Geronemus RG. Laser treatment in the management of infantile hemangiomas and capillary vascular malformations. Tech Vasc Interv Radiol 2013;16(1):51–4.
33. Park J, Yun SK, Cho YS, et al. Treatment of angiofibromas in tuberous sclerosis complex: the effect of topical rapamycin and concomitant laser therapy. Dermatology 2014;228(1):37–41.

34. Tieu DD, Ghodke BV, Vo NJ, et al. Single-stage excision of localized head and neck venous malformations using preoperative glue embolization. Otolaryngol Head Neck Surg 2013;148(4):678–84.
35. Murthy AS, Dawson A, Gupta D, et al. Utility and tolerability of the long-pulsed 1064-nm neodymium: yttrium-aluminum-garnet (LP Nd:YAG) laser for treatment of symptomatic or disfiguring vascular malformations in children and adolescents. J Am Acad Dermatol 2017;77(3):473–9.
36. Trost J, Buckley C, Smidt AC. Long-pulsed neodymium-doped yttrium aluminum garnet laser for glomuvenous malformations in adolescents. Pediatr Dermatol 2015;32(5):e217–8.
37. Savas JA, Ledon J, Franca K, et al. Carbon dioxide laser for the treatment of microcystic lymphatic malformations (lymphangioma circumscriptum): a systematic review. Dermatol Surg 2013;39(8):1147–57.
38. Shumaker PR, Dela Rosa KM, Krakowski AC. Treatment of lymphangioma circumscriptum using fractional carbon dioxide laser ablation. Pediatr Dermatol 2013;30(5):584–6 [Erratum appears in Pediatr Dermatol 2015;32(5):777].
39. Momen S, Mallipeddi R, Al-Niaimi F. The use of lasers in Becker's naevus: an evidence-based review. J Cosmet Laser Ther 2016;18(4):188–92.
40. Imayama S, Ueda S. Long- and short-term histological observations of congenital nevi treated with the normal-mode ruby laser. Arch Dermatol 1999; 135(10):1211–8.
41. Polubothu S, Kinsler VA. Final congenital melanocytic naevi colour is determined by normal skin colour and unaltered by superficial removal techniques: a longitudinal study. Br J Dermatol 2020;182(3):721–8.
42. Seo HM, Choi CW, Kim WS. Beneficial effects of early treatment of nevus of Ota with low-fluence 1,064-nm Q-switched Nd:YAG laser. Dermatol Surg 2015;41(1):142–8.
43. Yu P, Yu N, Diao W, et al. Comparison of clinical efficacy and complications between Q-switched alexandrite laser and Q-switched Nd:YAG laser on nevus of Ota: a systematic review and meta-analysis. Lasers Med Sci 2016;31(3):581–91.
44. Schoch JJ, Tollefson MM, Witman P, et al. Successful treatment of keratosis pilaris rubra with pulsed dye laser. Pediatr Dermatol 2016;33(4):443–6.
45. Lyons AB, Townsend SM, Turk D, et al. Laser and light-based treatment modalities for the management of hidradenitis suppurativa. Am J Clin Dermatol 2020;21:237–43.
46. Iranmanesh B, Khalili M, Zartab H, et al. Laser therapy in cutaneous and genital warts: a review article. Dermatol Ther 2021;34(1):e14671.
47. Maranda EL, Lim VM, Nguyen AH, et al. Laser and light therapy for facial warts: a systematic review. J Eur Acad Dermatol Venereol 2016;30(10):1700–7.
48. Krakowski, et al. Procedural pediatric dermatology. 1st edition. New York: Wolters Kluwer; 2021.
49. Yu W, Ma G, Qiu Y, et al. Why do port-wine stains (PWS) on the lateral face respond better to pulsed dye laser (PDL) than those located on the central face? J Am Acad Dermatol 2016;74(3):527–35.
50. Yu W, Zhu J, Han Y, et al. Assessment of outcomes with pulsed dye laser treatment of port-wine stains located proximally vs distally on extremities. JAMA Dermatol 2020;156(6):702–4.

Dermatologic Consequences of Substandard, Spurious, Falsely Labeled, Falsified, and Counterfeit Medications

Gabrielle H. Schwartzman, BS[a], Paige K. Dekker, MD[b], Anna S. Silverstein, MD[c], Natalia M. Fontecilla, MD[d], Scott A. Norton, MD, MPH, MSc[a,*]

KEYWORDS

- Counterfeit drugs • Drug eruptions • Substandard drugs • Fraud • Crime
- Pharmaceutical preparations

KEY POINTS

- Substandard and falsified medications are a global problem, leading the World Health Organization to estimate that up to 10% of medications worldwide are counterfeit, fraudulent, or falsely labeled.
- Quantitatively or qualitatively irregular pharmaceutical products affect individuals, families, communities, and entire populations by weakening primary prevention of disease and secondary containment of disease; permitting the rise of drug resistant pathogens; creating vulnerabilities to overdose or poisonings; and directly causing adverse reactions.
- One way for substandard or falsified medications to become available in the United States is via improper or illegal importation but it is often difficult to distinguish these products from authentic ones.
- Determining the cause of a suspected drug reaction is particularly challenging when the culprit is an unidentified and entirely unsuspected adulterant, contaminant, or substitution.

INTRODUCTION

The perception among most Americans is that federal agencies tightly regulate the production, packaging, distribution, and sale of pharmaceutical products. As a result, people generally believe that prescription medications are, for the most part, safe and effective. Admittedly, segments of the population may undergo temporal waves of uncertainty and suspicion, but this sort of hesitation usually dissipates under circumstances of dire illness.

Although generally favorable perceptions apply to medications regulated by federal agencies, many products, including dietary supplements and homeopathic remedies, are underregulated, and often come close to being unregulated.

Presented in part as an invited lecture at the International Congress of Pediatric Dermatology, July 2017, Chicago, IL.

[a] Department of Dermatology, George Washington University School of Medicine and Health Sciences, 2150 Pennsylvania Ave, NW, Suite 2B-430, Washington, DC 20037, USA; [b] Georgetown University School of Medicine, Washington, DC, USA; [c] University of North Carolina School of Medicine, Chapel Hill, NC, USA; [d] Department of Dermatology, Johns Hopkins Medicine, Baltimore, MD, USA
* Corresponding author.
E-mail address: scottanorton@gmail.com

Dermatol Clin 40 (2022) 227–236
https://doi.org/10.1016/j.det.2021.12.008
0733-8635/22/© 2021 Elsevier Inc. All rights reserved.

Table 1
Governing bodies differ in their classifications of counterfeit drugs

FDA[1]	Centers for Disease Control and Prevention[2]	WHO	Interpol[3]
Counterfeit/fake Spurious Substandard Falsified Falsely labeled	Counterfeit/fake	Substandard/out of specification Unregistered/unlicensed Falsified	Fake Stolen Illicit Counterfeit Falsified Diverted Smuggled Trafficked Expired

Current federal legislation enables many dietary supplements and homeopathic products to evade serious scrutiny for safety and efficacy.

In the United States, the Food and Drug Administration (FDA) and other agencies regulate safety and efficacy of pharmaceutical products and establish standards for manufacture or importation. Similarly, most nations and many international organizations have their own regulatory structures. But a parallel universe of fraudulent products, including treatments for common dermatologic conditions, exists with the *raison d'être* to evade the scrutiny and costs of regulatory adherence.

Nevertheless, some products, such as drugs and biologics that are fully regulated by federal agencies, may reach the public with various irregularities. In plain terms, two general types of irregularities exist: quantitative and qualitative. Quantitative irregularities manifest as either *too much* or *not enough* of the professed medication. Qualitative irregularities, however, are myriad and defy such simplification. Products can be contaminated, adulterated, substituted, or mislabeled, among other transgressions, all of which add to burdens of disease and costs to society. The World Health Organization (WHO) and the FDA have official terminologies to categorize counterfeit medications (**Table 1**). For example, the FDA uses the description *substandard, spurious, falsely labeled, falsified, and counterfeit (SSFFC) medical products*. Although the WHO uses different terminology, in this article we use SSFFC to encompass the entire range of products associated with some sort of fraud, deception, evasion, or criminality involved with bringing the product to public use.

In global pharmaceutical markets, the scale of counterfeit and otherwise fraudulent medications is staggering.[4] Approximately 10% of pharmaceutical products worldwide (approaching 30% in parts of Africa, Asia, and Latin America) are substandard in ways that are both lucrative and criminal. On a per use basis, fraudulent medications cause more adverse events than legitimate preparations and contribute to approximately 100,000 deaths/year worldwide. The entire problem is accelerating alongside the COVID-19-pandemic.[5]

All health care providers should be aware that these problems exist and also that they are increasing in the United States and abroad. The dermatology community has an important but ill-defined role in fighting this problem, especially by detecting suspicious products from their cutaneous side effects and then reporting the events. In this article, we describe the worldwide scope of the problem, discuss dermatologic consequences of such medications, and offer recommendations to help dermatologists respond to this public health issue.

Dermatologists in particular must be cognizant of the pervasive nature of SSFFC medications, given the frequency of cutaneous drug reactions and the extreme risks associated with severe drug reactions (eg, toxic epidermal necrolysis or drug reaction with eosinophilia and systemic symptoms). Determining the cause of a suspected drug reaction is particularly challenging when the culprit medication is an unidentified and entirely unsuspected adulterant, contaminant, or substitution.

Recognizing irregularities in the production of legitimate (ie, approved) drugs (as well as illicit drugs) is a public health issue of increasing importance, one that adds to the burdens of disease and costs to society. The introduction of counterfeit, contraband, and substandard medications can cause unanticipated adverse outcomes that affect the health of individuals, including untreated illnesses, prolonged suffering, drug overdose, adverse drug reactions, and death; but can also affect the health of populations by generating drug-resistant pathogens and failing to control the spread of disease.

In this article, we discuss SSFFC medications, the drug reactions they may cause, their effects on society, and ways to report possibly suspect products to the proper authorities. When possible, we emphasize aspects of the problem that affect children to conform to the scope of this special pediatric-focused issue of *Dermatologic Clinics*.

TERMINOLOGY

Until 2017, the WHO applied the label SSFFC for a wide range of medication irregularities.[4] In 2017, however, the WHO changed the collective label to substandard and falsified medical products[5] and created three subgroups: (1) substandard, (2) unregistered/unlicensed, and (3) falsified medical products (see **Table 1**).

Substandard, also called *out-of-specification*, products are "authorized medical products that fail to meet either their quality standards or their specifications, or both." *Unregistered/unlicensed* products are those that have "not undergone evaluation and/or approval by the National or Regional Regulatory Authority (NRRA) for the market in which they are marketed/distributed or used, subject to permitted conditions under national or regional regulation and legislation." Lastly, *falsified* medical products are those that "deliberately/fraudulently misrepresent their identity, composition or source." However, the FDA continues to use the WHO's older SSFFC terminology (**Table 2**).[1]

METHODS

To determine the extent and scope of the problem relating to dermatology worldwide (not just in the United States), we searched MEDLINE for examples of SSFFC products that were used to treat dermatologic conditions or that caused an adverse cutaneous drug reaction. Our goal was to find representative or instructive examples of each type of dermatology-related SSFFC category, not to exhaustively identify every documented case in the literature.

The key element in our search strategy was selecting MeSH terms that are associated with SSFFC medications. Using MeSH hierarchies available at www.ncbi.nlm.nih.gov/mesh/, we developed this strategy and searched via the OVID interface with MEDLINE, limiting the search to case reports and review articles published after 1946: *exp** (*exp* preceding a MeSH term indicates the term was used in its "exploded" form). Fraud/OR *exp* Prescription Drug Diversion/OR *exp* Substandard Drugs/OR *exp* Drug Trafficking/OR *exp* Counterfeit Drugs/OR *exp* Drug Contamination/OR Drug Industry/es,lj,st OR Pharmaceutical Preparations/st OR (*exp* Nonprescription Drugs/AND (Internet/OR Commerce/)). To narrow the list further, we used the Boolean AND function for (exp Dermatology/or exp Skin/or exp Skin Diseases/or exp Skin Neoplasms/or exp Skin Physiologic Phenomena/or exp Skin Manifestations/or exp Skin Abnormalities/).

Next, we examined the titles (and abstracts, if available) to identify relevant articles. We obtained and reviewed papers written in English, French, or

Table 2
Definitions as specified by the FDA[6]

Term	Definition
Substandard/out-of-specification	Products are proper pharmacologic products produced by manufacturers authorized by the National Medicines Regulatory Authority, although the specific products do not meet national quality specification standards.
Spurious drugs	Manufactured under a name of another drug, imitate another drug, or have been substituted wholly or partly by another drug. Spurious drugs thus conceal the true pharmacologic identity of the product or formulation. Spurious drugs generally resemble well-known brands in some way, but nevertheless conceal the true identity of the product or formulation.
Falsely labeled drugs	Genuine products with false packaging.
Falsified drugs	Produced criminally with fraudulent intent.
Counterfeit drugs	Drugs entail the deliberate attempt to imitate a genuine product; therefore, counterfeit medications are fakes intended to imitate a genuine product.[3]

Spanish. In addition, we perused each paper's list of references to uncover other potentially relevant publications.

RESULTS

Our search strategy produced a list of approximately 500 indexed papers, not all of which were relevant for the purpose of this article. We selected about 20% of the papers to review in detail and describe types of SSFFC-induced adverse effects in **Table 3**. In addition, we provide several instructive examples of dermatologic side effects of these products.

Case Study of Unregistered/Unlicensed Medications

One example involves cases of fixed drug eruptions caused by a contraband medication in a community of Salvadoran-American children in the Washington, DC, area. Several children presented with recurrences of unexplained blisters in fixed locations. We learned they had taken a

Table 3
Case examples of fraudulent medications (based on WHO classification)

Flaw in Medication	Example or Event	Consequence (Dermatologic or Other)	Location and Year
Substandard			
Bacterial contaminants	Desiccated placenta	Infant infection with Group B streptococci	Oregon, 2016[6]
Fungal contaminants	Methylprednisolone contaminated with fungi	Meningitis, epidural abscess, vertebral osteomyelitis, diskitis, phlegmon, arachnoiditis	Michigan, 2012–2013[7]
Heavy metals contaminants	Kelp supplements contaminated with arsenic	Memory loss, alopecia, rash, fatigue, debilitating nausea/vomiting	California, 2007[8]
Organic contaminants	L-tryptophan sleep supplements contaminated with di-tryptophan animal of acetaldehyde	Eosinophilia-myalgia syndrome	United States, 1985–1989[9]
Falsified			
Adulterated with corticosteroids	Topical steroids in Chinese cosmetics Clobetasol in "Asian herbal" compounds for atopic dermatitis Prescription-strength betamethasone purchased over the counter from African-wares store	Steroid-induced rosacea-like dermatitis Steroid atrophy Discontinued before adverse effects	China, 2017[10] Washington, DC, 2017[11]
Adulterated with antibiotics	Traveling peddlers selling medications containing cotrimoxazole	Fixed drug eruption	Republic of Congo, 2005–2008[12]
Unregistered/unlicensed			
Medication licensed abroad but not in United States	Baczol cold medication containing cotrimoxazole	Fixed drug eruption	Washington, DC, 2017[13]
Preparations purchased online	Bleaching creams	Chemical burns	California, 2015[14]

cough and cold medication called Baczol Antigripal[13] manufactured in El Salvador. The product contains a sulfonamide antibiotic, trimethoprim-sulfamethoxazole, which is available over the counter in El Salvador but requires a prescription in the United States. Although the box stated (in Spanish) that sale was permitted only in El Salvador and required a prescription, the patient's families bought these products without prescriptions at Hispanic grocery stores in the Washington, DC, area.

In 2013, a team investigated the availability of Baczol products and found them for sale without prescription in 7 of 19 Hispanic grocery stores in DC, Maryland, and Virginia, despite an existing FDA import alert that prohibited their sale in the United States. Trimethoprim-sulfamethoxazole has many serious adverse effects including toxic epidermal necrolysis, Stevens-Johnson syndrome, nephrotoxicity, bone marrow suppression, and benign cutaneous hypersensitivity and photosensitivity reactions.

Case Study of Falsified Medications

Patients may develop signs of topical steroid overuse after treating such conditions as atopic dermatitis with adulterated products. For example, many patients at the pediatric dermatology clinic at Birmingham (UK) Children's Hospital reported good results from treating their atopic eczema with over-the-counter "herbal creams." The investigators analyzed 24 creams submitted by 19 patients and found clobetasol propionate, clobetasone butyrate, betamethasone valerate, and other potent-to-ultrapotent corticosteroids in the purportedly "herbal" products.[15]

Another report describes the pervasive presence of topical steroids in Chinese cosmetics.[10] These adulterated preparations, marketed as safe herbal folk remedies, can lead to serious dermatologic and systemic complications.

Finding products labeled as "herbal" but adulterated with pharmaceuticals and even with animal parts (quite the opposite of herbal) is well-described. One paper describes a nationally distributed "herbal" product whose label listed 17 bovine organs among its ingredients, including brain, spleen, lung, liver, pancreas, pituitary, pineal gland, adrenal glands, lymph node, placenta, prostate, heart, kidney, and intestine.[16,17] That paper suggests that customers may be unfamiliar with, and therefore misunderstand, ingredient names, such as orchis, which means the substance was derived from testicles, not orchids. Nevertheless, the product was sold at a nationwide chain as an "herbal" dietary supplement.

These examples of products labeled as "natural" yet containing ingredients ranging from bovine testicles to illegal amphetamines, highlight the medical and social implications of such adulterated products. Consumers should be reminded that products marked as "natural supplements" are often wrongly perceived as inherently benign and therefore dismissed by the public as "safe" and free of potent drugs and medications.

Case Study of a "Nonexistent" Medication

Paradoxically, the absence of an expected medication can lead to cutaneous adverse events. An instance of a reaction caused by a "nonexistent" medication arose in preterm infants born less than 24-week gestation, who developed unexplained erosions (on perianal and perioral surfaces) and blisters (on dorsal hands and feet).[18] All affected infants were on total parenteral nutrition that was later determined to lack supplemental zinc, leading to a classic presentation of zinc-deficiency disorder. This situation was the consequence of a national shortage of injectable, sterile, parenteral-grade zinc that is a necessary component of complete parenteral nutrition preparations. The observation was reported to the FDA, who issued an immediate nationwide alert. The Centers for Disease Control and Prevention found similar cases at other neonatal intensive care units; however, the problem was soon corrected with restoration of the supply of parenteral-grade zinc.[18]

Case Study of a Substandard Medication

Commercially available medications and supplements may not always meet quality specifications set forth by regulatory agencies. For example, a 54-year-old woman presented to an occupational medicine clinic with a 2-year history of alopecia and memory loss.[8] A urine sample revealed an arsenic level of 83.6 μg/g of urinary creatinine (normal <50 μg/g creatinine). Her symptoms were caused by arsenic-contaminated kelp supplements, which she took daily. The investigative team then measured arsenic levels in several commercially available kelp supplements and found arsenic levels exceeding FDA limits in eight of nine samples obtained from local health stores.[8] The case report did not comment on the source or reason for the contamination. Other published reports indicate that arsenic-contaminated dietary supplements are manufactured most commonly in China or other East Asian nations, which is similar to the situation with a vast range of products contaminated with heavy metals .

These examples represent some of the dermatologic problems associated with SSFFC products. **Table 3** provides a more comprehensive list to give a more complete perspective of the scope of the problem and some of its clinical implications.

DISCUSSION

Substandard and falsified medical products and medications are a global problem. The WHO estimates that up to 10% of medications worldwide are counterfeit; this figure may be 30% in parts of Africa, Asia, and Latin America.[19] Moreover, most online or Internet-based pharmacies are noncompliant with federal, state, or industry standards, and many countries lack a rigorously functioning pharmaceutical regulatory agency. Counterfeit medications generate an estimated $75 billion in annual revenue and cause up to 100,000 deaths worldwide each year.[20]

Scope of the Problem in Dermatology

Adverse events associated with counterfeit medications are inevitable. **Table 3** lists additional adverse dermatologic side effects, ranging from chemical burns, skin abscesses, alopecia, and fixed drug eruptions attributed to counterfeit pharmaceuticals.

The scope of counterfeit medications in dermatology also includes substandard, fraudulent, and unlicensed dermatologic drugs and treatments. For example, four patients in Florida developed botulism after cosmetic injections with unlicensed botulinum preparation.[21] The injections contained 3000 times the estimated fatal toxin dose. This example shows that unlicensed botulinum products can cause serious illness and highlights need for strict compliance with (or enforcement of) existing regulations.

Illicit or unregulated products can cause adverse health outcomes. Illicit cosmetic fillers have caused several deaths,[22] leading to an awareness campaign by the American Society of Plastic Surgeons.[22] Cases include a 35-year-old transsexual woman presenting to an emergency room with tachypnea, tachycardia, and cyanosis. The patient was in shock after receiving multiple subcutaneous gluteal injections of polymethyl methacrylate (PMMA) microspheres.[23] Because of the patient's history of PMMA injections 4 days earlier, along with the absence of infectious signs, such as fever or blood culture growth, the authors hypothesize that the PMMA induced the systemic inflammatory response syndrome. Another case details a 66-year-old woman who developed heart failure and an inflammatory reaction after illegal cosmetic injections of PMMA or polyacrylamide hydrogel.[24]

Mesotherapy is intended to improve one's overall appearance of health and to decrease signs of aging by promoting lipolysis through subcutaneous injections of preparations containing vitamins and natural plant extracts.[25] One form of mesotherapy is FDA-approved for decreasing submental fat but many others, often marketed as "biorejuvenation," are legal in parts of South America and Europe, but illegal in the United States. Mesotherapy can involve injection of various substances, ranging from off-label use of approved injectable medications to homemade "herbal" preparations including bile acids, caffeine, and plant extracts. Adverse effects of injection with unregulated substances range from noninfectious suppurative panniculitis[26] to cutaneous tuberculosis[27] and are well-reported in the literature.

Bacterial contamination of injected medications and diluents is another hazard of irregularly prepared products. Infection with atypical mycobacteria is a well-described consequence of improper injection practices or nonsterile diluents.[28] A niche but telling example: the presence of postinjection abscesses and granulomas in children adopted from orphanages in Russia and other former Soviet states.[29]

According to the adoptive parents, the orphanages want children adopted from their facilities to arrive in their new homes healthy, infection-free, and with robust appetites. Therefore, the children were injected with vitamins and prescription medications, allegedly antibiotics "to prevent infections" and possibly glucocorticoids "to increase the child's appetite when the family arrives at the new home." Oftentimes, children receive injections of vaccines, vitamins, and medications that may be unnecessary or administered with improper technique. The injected products may be prepared with nonsterile diluents, such as tap water, which often contain atypical mycobacteria living in the biofilm of the water taps. Indurated lesions at injection sites, often the upper-outer buttocks, of these children may represent infections, hematomas, reactions to vaccine adjuvants, and/or sterile abscesses.

Scope of the Problem Beyond Dermatology

Substandard and falsified medications appear in almost every area of medicine and have staggering effects on the health of individuals and populations. Particularly egregious examples include false vaccines, completely devoid of antigenic material, distributed in China[30]; counterfeit or substandard antimalarials in South East Asia[31,32];

and contraceptive pills in Brazil that contain only starch and thus had no hormonal action.[33] These examples can have significant consequences, some of which are obvious (eg, unplanned pregnancies in the case of bogus oral contraceptives) and some less apparent (eg, vulnerability to vaccine-preventable diseases in the case of ersatz vaccines).

Manufacturers of counterfeit pharmaceuticals use sophisticated techniques to make their products nearly indistinguishable from authentic agents. A team investigating health-related crimes in Southeast Asia found that substandard artesunate, sold to treat malaria, was packaged in boxes with fraudulent holograms, designed to resemble proper packages of authentic artesunate.[32] Another report describes online-purchased counterfeit sildenafil arriving with individual capsules secure in seemingly genuine blister packets but packaged with falsified company logos and stamped with phony lot numbers.[34,35]

In many countries, national regulatory authorities permit over-the-counter sale of antibacterial and antimalarial agents. Frequent use, often without medical indication or in the wrong dose and duration, contributes to antimicrobial resistance. In India, several oral and parenteral antibiotics (eg, gentamicin, piperacillin-tazobactam, linezolid, and tigecycline) are approved for use but are not included in the national drug schedule and are therefore available without prescription.[36]

A Centers for Disease Control and Prevention study released in 2016 found that US-based dermatologists prescribe antibiotics at rates higher than any other specialty.[37] There is concern that dermatologists overprescribe antibiotics, especially when written for prophylaxis of perioperative infections.[38,39] Therefore, dermatologists may be unwitting contributors to widespread antibiotic resistance. This consequence is presumably more pronounced in countries where antibiotics are not tightly regulated and where fraudulent antibiotics are commonly sold.

Monitoring and detecting potentially fraudulent behaviors and practices is difficult, time-consuming, and costly. As a result, the world of fraudulent and counterfeit medications is unmonitored, which lowers the risk of intervention by law enforcement, making the enterprise especially attractive to organized crime.

The pharmaceutical supply chain is multistepped and complex. Many steps are vulnerable to corruption, from obtaining base materials; manufacturing the active ingredients; and storing, transporting, and distributing product. The expansion of Internet pharmacies further complicates the task of monitoring the distribution and sale of counterfeit medications.[19]

The production and sale of counterfeit, substandard, and missing medications is a profitable endeavor, especially when specific drugs are in short supply. Drug counterfeiters can take advantage of a high-demand market by charging exorbitant prices.[19] For example, during a brief period in 2011, drugs in short supply had price markups averaging 650% and soared up to 4533% for labetalol.[40]

Penalties for engaging in these activities are weak or nonexistent. The criminal penalties associated with illegally sale of narcotics are much higher than those associated with the sale of counterfeit drugs.[19]

Many organizations, governmental and nongovernmental, are taking steps to address the problems associated with SSFFC products (**Box 1**). In this regard the International Coalition of Medicines Regulatory Authorities provides "a global architecture to support enhanced communication, information sharing, crisis response and address regulatory science issues."[43] The FDA and regulatory agencies for most European countries and developed nations worldwide are members of the International Coalition of Medicines Regulatory Authorities.

The International Police (Interpol) and the Medicines and Healthcare Products Regulatory Agency of the WHO manage a program called Operation Pangaea. This is an annual week-long event that addresses the online sale of counterfeit and illicit pharmaceuticals. Since its launch in 2008, participation in Operation Pangaea has grown from 10 countries to more than 100. The results include seizure of 21-million units of fake and illicit medicines, more than 150 arrests, launching more than 400 investigations, removing hundreds of Internet advertisements for illicit pharmaceuticals, and shutting down greater than 2400 Web sites.[44]

The United States has also taken legislative action. President Barack Obama signed the Drug Quality and Security Act into law in 2013, allowing secure tracing of medical products from manufacturer to pharmacy. This track-and-trace system makes it difficult for counterfeit drugs to enter the legitimate pharmaceutical supply chain.[19] Successfully combatting this problem requires continued collaboration among governments, law enforcement agencies, pharmaceutical industries, and the public.

Helping patients avoid adverse side effects from counterfeit medications also requires participation of providers in all medical fields. Providers are becoming more accustomed to asking patients about over-the-counter medications, herbal and

Box 1
Steps to take with suspected substandard or falsified products

Reporting to the FDA[41]

To report a life-threatening situation caused by an FDA-regulated product online or in store, first call 911, then call 1-866-300-4374, the FDA emergency hotline.

As a consumer or health care professional, if you believe that you have a suspect counterfeit drug, report it to the FDA's MedWatch Office (www.fda.gov/Safety/MedWatch) and contact the pharmacy or company from where the drug was purchased.

If you suspect that a Web site is selling counterfeit drugs, report it to the FDA (www.fda.gov/Safety/ReportaProblem/ucm059315.htm). If you purchase drugs from an online pharmacy, make sure that it is one of the Verified Internet Pharmacy Practice Sites (VIPPS) accredited through the National Association of Boards of Pharmacy.

If you are aware of suspicious activities associated with counterfeit drugs, report it to the FDA's Office of Criminal Investigations (www.accessdata.fda.gov/scripts/email/oc/oci/contact.cfm).

Reporting to the WHO[42]

If you think a product you have used is a substandard or falsified product, report it to the WHO via their rapid report system. The WHO will investigate the claim, and if the threat is validated and poses a harm to public health, a Medical Product Rapid Alert will be issued (www.who.int/medicines/regulation/ssffc/medical-products/en/).

Reporting to Interpol

To contact Interpol to inquire about possible pharmaceutical crime, you may fill out an inquiry form from their Web site (www.interpol.int/Forms/Pharmaceutical_crime). This is not a tracking or reporting system. Reports should be directed to the FDA or WHO, agencies that then share collected information with Interpol to coordinate responses.

dietary supplements, and so forth. Providers should also ask patients about medications obtained abroad, received from family members abroad, or that may have been brought into the United States illegally ("unsupervised importation") and subsequently sold (eg, in ethnic markets and shops).

All physicians should be aware of problems associated with fraudulent medications; dermatologists must remember that fraudulent medications, just like authentic ones, can cause cutaneous adverse reactions. In general, when physicians evaluate a suspected drug eruption, their cognitive process starts by matching lesional morphology with the medication classes to which the patient has been exposed. This line of inquiry is difficult, however, when the culprit medication is an unidentified and unsuspected adulterant, contaminant, or substitution.

Counterfeit drugs comprise a growing percentage of the pharmaceutical market in the United States, and an even greater percentage in developing countries, many of which lack a well-functioning pharmaceutical regulatory agency.[19] Moreover, most online pharmacies are noncompliant with federal, state, or industry standards. Although this is a growing public health concern worldwide, consumers are largely unaware of the spectrum of consequences associated with fraudulent medications.

Fraudulent medications interfere with the treatment of individual medical concerns, with primary prevention of disease, with secondary containment of disease, with maintaining or improving health, with limiting the spread of drug-resistant pathogens, with potential overdosing or poisoning, with direct adverse reactions, and with drug-drug interactions. These consequences affect individuals, families, communities, and entire populations.

CLINICS CARE POINTS

- A thorough medication history will include questions about medications obtained abroad, received from family members abroad, brought into the United States as an "unsupervised importation", or that were obtained at internet pharmacies or ethnic markets and shops.
- Substandard medications can enter the supply chain at many points, eg, manufacture, packaging, importation, distribution, storage, dispensing, and sale.
- Do not use products, even cosmetic ones, that are imported illegally or possibly produced under fraudulent or substandard circumstances.
- Mechanisms to report possible substandard medications to the Food and Drug Administration are straightforward and an essential part of maintaining the health of individual paitients, their families, the local community, and the public at large.

FINANCIAL DISCLOSURE STATEMENT

There are no financial disclosures, commercial associations, or any other conditions posing a conflict of interest to report for any of the authors.

REFERENCES

1. United States Food and Drug Administration. Counterfeit medicine. Available at: https://www.fda.gov/drugs/buying-using-medicine-safely/counterfeit-medicine. Accessed July 7, 2020.
2. Centers for Disease Control and Prevention. Counterfeit medicines. Available at: https://wwwnc.cdc.gov/travel/page/counterfeit-medicine. Accessed July 7, 2020.
3. Interpol. Fake Medicines. Available at: https://www.interpol.int/en/Crimes/Illicit-goods/Shop-safely/Fake-medicines. Accessed July 7, 2020.
4. World Health Organization. Definitions of substandard and falsified (SF) medical products. Available at: https://www.who.int/medicines/regulation/ssffc/definitions/en/. Accessed June 6, 2020.
5. Olliaro E, Olliaro P, Ho CWL, et al. Legal uncertainty - The gray area around substandard medicines: where public health meets law. Am J Trop Med Hyg 2020;102(2):262–7. https://doi.org/10.4269/ajtmh.19-0645.
6. Buser GL, Mató S, Zhang AY, et al. Late-onset infant group B Streptococcus infection associated with maternal consumption of capsules containing dehydrated placenta—Oregon, 2016. MMWR Morb Mortal Wkly Rep 2017;66(25):677–8. https://doi.org/10.15585/mmwr.mm6625a4.
7. Centers for Disease Control. Spinal and paraspinal infections associated with contaminated methylprednisolone acetate injections—Michigan, 2012-2013. MMWR Morb Mortal Wkly Rep 2013;62(19):377–81.
8. Amster E, Tiwary A, Schenker MB. Case report: Potential arsenic toxicosis secondary to herbal kelp supplement. Environ Health Perspect 2007;115(4):606–8. https://doi.org/10.1289/ehp.9495.
9. Centers for Disease Control and Prevention. Update: analysis of L-tryptophan for the etiology of eosinophilia-myalgia syndrome. MMWR Morb Mortal Wkly Rep 1990;39(43):789–90.
10. Xie H, Xiao X, Li J. Topical steroids in Chinese cosmetics. JAMA Dermatol 2017;153(9):855–6. https://doi.org/10.1001/jamadermatol.2017.1615.
11. Burke KT, Fricke MA, DeKlotz CMC. Prescription-strength topical steroids sold without prescription. JAMA Dermatol 2017;153(12):1337–8. https://doi.org/10.1001/jamadermatol.2017.4121.
12. Ognongo-Ibiaho AN, Atanda HL. Epidemiological study of fixed drug eruption in Pointe-Noire. Int J Dermatol 2012;51(Suppl 1):30–5. https://doi.org/10.1111/j.1365-4632.2012.05561.x.
13. Yang CC, Green AN, Norton SA. Fixed drug eruption associated with sulfonamides sold in Latino grocery stores—greater Washington, DC, Area, 2012-2013. MMWR Morb Mortal Wkly Rep 2013;62(46):914–6.
14. Totri CR, Diaz L, Matiz C, et al. A 15-year-old girl with painful, peeling skin. Pediatr Ann 2015;44(5):195–7. https://doi.org/10.3928/00904481-20150512-06.
15. Ramsay HM, Goddard W, Gill S, et al. Herbal creams used for atopic eczema in Birmingham, UK illegally contain potent corticosteroids. Arch Dis Child 2003;88(12):1056–7. https://doi.org/10.1136/adc.88.12.1056.
16. Norton SA. Raw animal tissues and dietary supplements. N Engl J Med 2000;343(4):304–5. https://doi.org/10.1056/NEJM200007273430417.
17. Cohen PA. American roulette: contaminated dietary supplements. N Engl J Med 2009;361(16):1523–5. https://doi.org/10.1056/NEJMp0904768.
18. Ruktanonchai D, Lowe M, Norton SA, et al. Zinc deficiency-associated dermatitis in infants during a nationwide shortage of injectable zinc—Washington, DC, and Houston, TX, 2012-2013. MMWR Morb Mortal Wkly Rep 2014;63(2):35–7.
19. Blackstone EA, Fuhr JP, Pociask S. The health and economic effects of counterfeit drugs. Am Heal Drug Benefits 2014;7(4):216–24.
20. Wechsler J. Campaign mounts to curb counterfeit drugs: manufacturers and regulators struggle to control phony versions of crucial medicines. Biopharm Int 2012;25(9):14.
21. Chertow DS, Tan ET, Maslanka SE, et al. Botulism in 4 adults following cosmetic injections with an unlicensed, highly concentrated botulinum preparation. J Am Med Assoc 2006;296(20):2476–9. https://doi.org/10.1001/jama.296.20.2476.
22. Leonardi NR, Compoginis JM, Luce EA. Illicit cosmetic silicone injection: a recent reiteration of history. Ann Plast Surg 2016;77(4):485–90. https://doi.org/10.1097/SAP.0000000000000756.
23. Boattini M, Francisco AR, Cavaco R, et al. Shock following subcutaneous injections of polymethylmethacrylate. Med Intensiva 2015;39(4):256–7. https://doi.org/10.1016/j.medin.2014.06.011.
24. Purnell CA, Klosowiak JL, Cheesborough JE, et al. Resolution of cosmetic buttock injection-induced inflammatory reaction and heart failure after excision of filler material. Plast Reconstr Surg Glob Open 2016;4(10):e1079. https://doi.org/10.1097/GOX.0000000000001079.
25. El-Domyati M, El-Ammawi TS, Moawad O, et al. Efficacy of mesotherapy in facial rejuvenation: a histological and immunohistochemical evaluation. Int J Dermatol 2012;51(8):913–9. https://doi.org/10.1111/j.1365-4632.2011.05184.x.

26. Campos LM, Miot LDB, Marques MEA, et al. Case for diagnosis. Noninfectious suppurative panniculitis induced by mesotherapy with deoxycholate. An Bras Dermatol 2019;94(6):754–6. https://doi.org/10.1016/j.abd.2019.02.003.
27. Orjuela D, Puerto G, Mejía G, et al. Cutaneous tuberculosis after mesotherapy: report of six cases [Tuberculosis cutánea por mesoterapia, estudio de seis casos]. Biomedica 2010;30(3):321.
28. Yuan J, Liu Y, Yang Z, et al. Mycobacterium abscessus post-injection abscesses from extrinsic contamination of multiple-dose bottles of normal saline in a rural clinic. Int J Infect Dis 2009;13(5):537–42. https://doi.org/10.1016/j.ijid.2008.11.024.
29. Kimes K, Marchalik R, Aivaz O, et al. Postinjection abscesses and granulomas in children adopted from Russia. Pediatr Dermatol 2019;36(4):e93–4. https://doi.org/10.1111/pde.13835.
30. McLaughlin K. Scandal clouds China's global vaccine ambitions. Science 2016;352(6285):506. https://doi.org/10.1126/science.352.6285.506.
31. Lon CT, Tsuyuoka R, Phanouvong S, et al. Counterfeit and substandard antimalarial drugs in Cambodia. Trans R Soc Trop Med Hyg 2006; 100(11):1019–114. https://doi.org/10.1016/j.trstmh.2006.01.003.
32. Newton PN, Fernández FM, Plançon A, et al. A collaborative epidemiological investigation into the criminal fake artesunate trade in South East Asia. Plos Med 2008;5(2):e32. https://doi.org/10.1371/journal.pmed.0050032.
33. BBC News. Brazil's bitter pill. 1998. Available at: http://news.bbc.co.uk/2/hi/americas/123741.stm. Accessed Jnauary 14, 2022.
34. Campbell N, Clark JP, Stecher VJ, et al. Internet-ordered Viagra (sildenafil citrate) is rarely genuine. J Sex Med 2012;9(11):2943–51. https://doi.org/10.1111/j.1743-6109.2012.02877.x.
35. Lehmann A, Katerere DR, Dressman J. Drug quality in South Africa: a field test. J Pharm Sci 2018; 107(10):2720–30. https://doi.org/10.1016/j.xphs.2018.06.012.
36. Laxminarayan R, Chaudhury RR. Antibiotic resistance in India: drivers and opportunities for action. PLoS Med 2016;13(3):e1001974. https://doi.org/10.1371/journal.pmed.1001974.
37. Centers for Disease Control and Prevention. Outpatient antibiotic prescriptions: United States, 2016. Available at: https://www.cdc.gov/antibiotic-use/community/pdfs/Annual-Report-2016-H.pdf. Accessed July 7, 2020.
38. Bae-Harboe YSC, Liang CA. Perioperative antibiotic use of dermatologic surgeons in 2012. Dermatol Surg 2013;39(11):1592–601. https://doi.org/10.1111/dsu.12272.
39. Barbieri JS, Bhate K, Hartnett KP, et al. Trends in oral antibiotic prescription in dermatology, 2008 to 2016. JAMA Dermatol 2019;155(3):290–7. https://doi.org/10.1001/jamadermatol.2018.4944.
40. Cherici C, McGinnis P, Russell W. Buyer beware: drug shortages and the gray market. Premier healthcare alliance report 2011. Available at: https://www.premierinc.com/about/news/11-aug/Gray-Market/Gray-Market-Analysis-08152011.pdf. Accessed July 7, 2020.
41. United States Food and Drug Administration. What should I do if I believe I have received or taken counterfeit medicine? Information for consumers and health providers. Available at: https://www.fda.gov/drugs/counterfeit-medicine/what-should-i-do-if-i-believe-i-have-received-or-taken-counterfeit-medicine-information-consumers. Accessed July 7, 2020.
42. World Health Organization. WHO medical product alerts – background. Available at: https://www.who.int/medicines/regulation/ssffc/medical-products/en/. Accessed July 7, 2020.
43. International Coalition of Medicines Regulatory Authorities (ICMRA). International Coalition of Medicines Regulatory Authorities (ICMRA). Available at: http://www.icmra.info/drupal/en/home. Accessed July 7, 2020.
44. Interpol. INTERPOL-coordinated operation strikes at organized crime with seizure of 20 million illicit medicines. 2015. Available at: https://www.interpol.int/en/News-and-Events/News/2015/INTERPOL-coordinated-operation-strikes-at-organized-crime-with-seizure-of-20-million-illicit-medicines. Accessed July 7, 2020.

Moving?

Make sure your subscription moves with you!

To notify us of your new address, find your **Clinics Account Number** (located on your mailing label above your name), and contact customer service at:

Email: journalscustomerservice-usa@elsevier.com

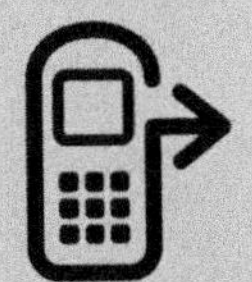

800-654-2452 (subscribers in the U.S. & Canada)
314-447-8871 (subscribers outside of the U.S. & Canada)

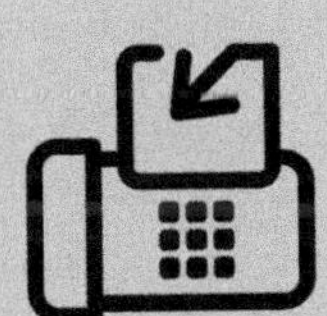

Fax number: 314-447-8029

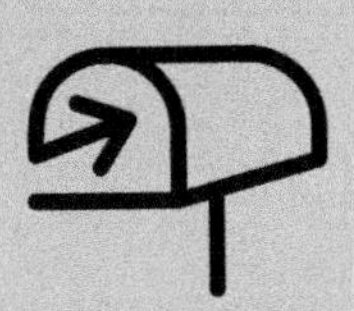

Elsevier Health Sciences Division
Subscription Customer Service
3251 Riverport Lane
Maryland Heights, MO 63043

*To ensure uninterrupted delivery of your subscription, please notify us at least 4 weeks in advance of move.

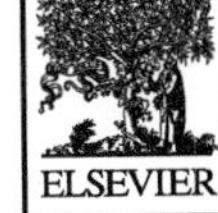

Printed and bound by CPI Group (UK) Ltd, Croydon, CR0 4YY
08/05/2025
01864713-0013